Dental Care and Oral Health

Dental Care and Oral Health

Edited by Victor Martinez

hayle medical

New York

Hayle Medical,
750 Third Avenue, 9ᵗʰ Floor,
New York, NY 10017, USA

Visit us on the World Wide Web at:
www.haylemedical.com

ISBN: 978-1-63241-563-9

Trademark Notice: Registered trademark of products or corporate names are used only for explanation and identification without intent to infringe.

Cataloging-in-Publication Data

Dental care and oral health / edited by Victor Martinez.
    p. cm.
Includes bibliographical references and index.
ISBN 978-1-63241-563-9
1. Dental care. 2. Mouth--Care and hygiene. 3. Oral medicine. 4. Dental hygiene.
5. Dental public health. 6. Mouth--Diseases. 7. Dentistry. I. Martinez, Victor.
RK58 .D46 2019
617.600 68--dc23

Table of Contents

Preface

Dentistry is a branch of medicine that deals with dental care and oral health. It also studies the diseases and disorders of the oral cavity. The medical conditions of the adjacent tissues and other structures related to the oral cavity are also studied under this branch of medicine. The temporomandibular joint and its supporting muscular, nervous, vascular and anatomical structures are of particular interest in this field. Tooth decay is a common disease. Restorative dental treatments include fillings, crowns and bridges, whereas, prosthetic treatments include removable or fixed dentures. This book elucidates the concepts and innovative models around prospective developments with respect to dental care and oral health. It includes some of the vital pieces of work being conducted across the world, on various topics related to dental care and oral health. The extensive content of this book provides the readers with a thorough understanding of the subject.

The information contained in this book is the result of intensive hard work done by researchers in this field. All due efforts have been made to make this book serve as a complete guiding source for students and researchers. The topics in this book have been comprehensively explained to help readers understand the growing trends in the field.

I would like to thank the entire group of writers who made sincere efforts in this book and my family who supported me in my efforts of working on this book. I take this opportunity to thank all those who have been a guiding force throughout my life.

Editor

1

Early Treatment of Anterior Crossbite Relating to Functional Class III

Sanaa Alami, Hakima Aghoutan, Farid El Quars,
Samir Diouny and Farid Bourzgui

1. Introduction

Anterior crossbite is one of the most common orthodontic problems observed in children's growth, in both skeletal and functional Class III malocclusion. The latter presents an apparent imbalance in jaw size, considered to be essentially the result of a mesial thrust of the mandible. Its origins are multiple, ranging from abnormal eruption of deciduous or definitive incisors to lingual dysfunction (low position of the tongue) [1].

Functional Class III has long-term effects on the growth and development of the teeth. This widely justifies the need for early treatment to normalize the occlusion and create conditions for normal jaws development. An accurate diagnosis is required for successful treatment and stability.

Orthodontists must distinguish pseudo Class III crossbites from skeletal Class III. Thorough clinical assessment and accurate diagnosis must be performed in order to plan proper treatment strategies and appliance design during the early stages of dental development. In this respect, various modes of treatment have been suggested for anterior crossbite correction [2, 3, 4, 5]; early interceptive treatment is one mode of treatment, which has been suggested because of its diverse benefits.

This chapter aims (1) to define functional mandibular prognathism and its etiopathogeny, (2) to highlight the needs to manage earlier anterior crossbites, and finally (3) to illustrate the impact of interceptive approach with the use of a simple fixed appliance.

2. Functional mandibular prognathism

The functional mandibular prognathism referred as mandibular pseudo-prognathism, or pseudo-Class III, is a mandibular abnormal function belonging to the class III malocclusion according to the terminology of Angle [1, 6]. The aforementioned is an anomaly of occlusal origin, which develops into a skeletal anomaly (true Class III). Indeed, the functional disorder translates into a normal closure until the premature contact [7].

Anterior crossbite is defined as a situation in which one or more permanent mandibular incisors occlude labially to their antagonists [4], which can be associated or not to a mandibular lateral-deviation [7].

2.1. Etiopathogeny

Pseudo-Class III malocclusion is identified as an anterior crossbite as a result of mandibular displacement. The reported prevalence of anterior crossbites varies between 2.2% and 12%, depending on children's age and their ethnicity [2, 8, 9, 10].

Moyers suggested that pseudo-Class III malocclusion was a positional relationship related to an acquired neutomuscular reflex. The anterior crossbite that results is established in the mixed dentition. Different etiological factors are involved; they can be classified in dental, functional and skeletal factors [4, 8, 9].

Dental factors:

- Palatal eruption of the maxillary central incisors,

- Proclination of the lower incisors due to low thrust lingual or supernumerary anterior teeth in mandible,

- Premature loss of the the primary upper incisors following a dental trauma,

- Over-retained primary maxillary incisors due to odontomas,

- Crowding in the incisor region, and inadequate arch length

Functional factors:

- Tongue position anomalies

- Nasorespiratory problems

Skeletal factors:

- Minor transverse maxillary discrepancy.

Premature contact between the maxillary and mandibular incisors results in a forward displacement of the mandible to permit a comfortably occlusion [4, 9, 11].

2.2. Prognosis

Functional mandibular prognathism in the early mixed dentition can have long-term effects on the growth and development of the teeth and jaws (McNamara, 2002). Anterior crossbite may lead to abnormal enamel abrasion or proclination of the mandibular incisors, which, in turn, leads to gingival recession. Abnormal mandibular shift caused by lack of incisal guide may have adverse effects on the temporo-mandibular joints and masticatory system [4, 12].

What is most to be feared is that a functional anomaly becomes a skeletal prognathism. Indeed, spontaneous correction of such malocclusion has been reported to be too low to justify non-intervention. Therefore, interceptive treatment is often advised to normalize the occlusion and create conditions for normal occlusal development [4].

3. Diagnostic approach

Class III malocclusion has been divided into two subtypes: Skeletal and pseudo-Class III [5]. The early management of the pseudo-class III presents no real difficulties. Timing and modalities of treatment depend on the differential diagnosis which aims to determine whether the crossbite is dental or skeletal in nature. An essential aspect of the differential diagnosis in Class III malocclusion is the assessment of dental compensations and the presence of functional slide via a thorough clinical and radiographic analysis [13].

3.1. Clinical analysis

3.1.1. Exobuccal evaluation

Exobuccal signs are practically the same for both types of dysmorphia (skeletal and functional Class III) which are, most of the time, misleading. There is usually a concave profile, characterized by an inversion of the labial relationship as well as a projection at the front of the mandibule (Figure 1). Usually, soft tissues tend to camouflage skeletal discrepancy so that the patient's profile appears normal or slightly concave in centric occlusion (Figure 2) [10].

It is important to note that although skeletal Class III is mandibular or maxillary, there is some degree of maxillary deficiency. Skeletal Class III, therefore, differs by a retrusive nasomaxillary area, and an important protrusive lower face and lip (Figure 3) [14].

The clinical assessment of profile changes from postural rest position to habitual occlusion is an additional criterion to be evaluated. The skeletal Class III profile remains concave in both positions, whereas the pseudo-class III profile is usually straight, but becomes concave as the mandible shifts forward into habitual occlusion position [9]. As many signs, which could mislead to a true Class III diagnosis.

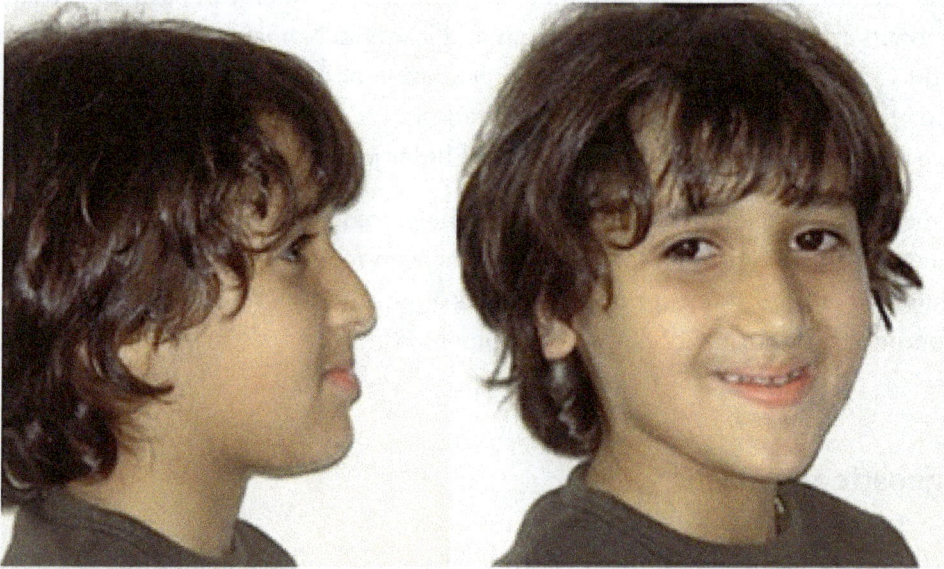

Figure 1. A patient, aged 8, presents pseudo-Class III malocclusion characterized by retrusion of the upper lip relative to the lower lip; smile betrays an anterior crossbite

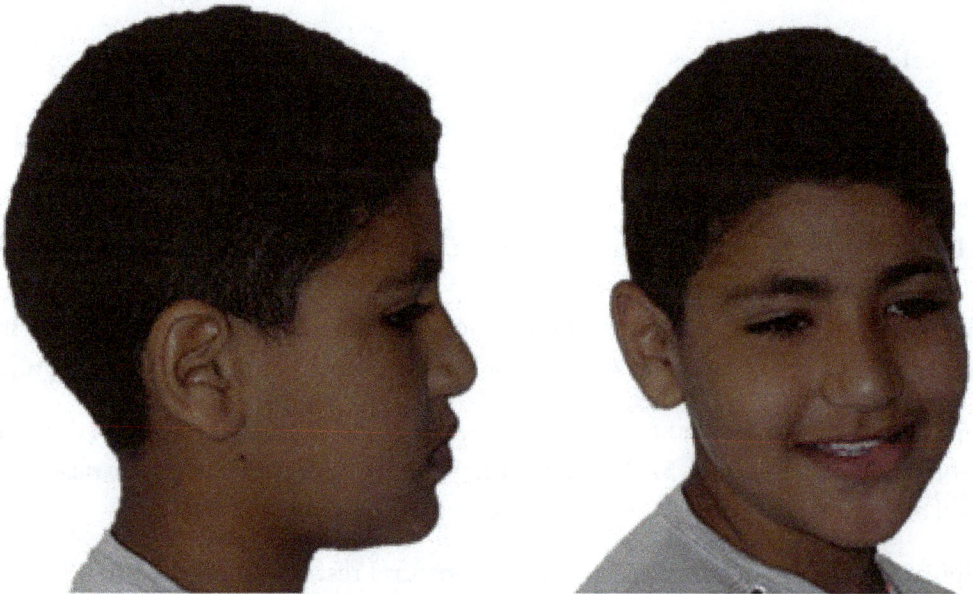

Figure 2. A patient, aged 9, presents pseudo-Class III malocclusion and a convex soft-tissue profile; labial relationships appear normal. Anterior cross-bite is revealed only on the views of smiling face and ¾.

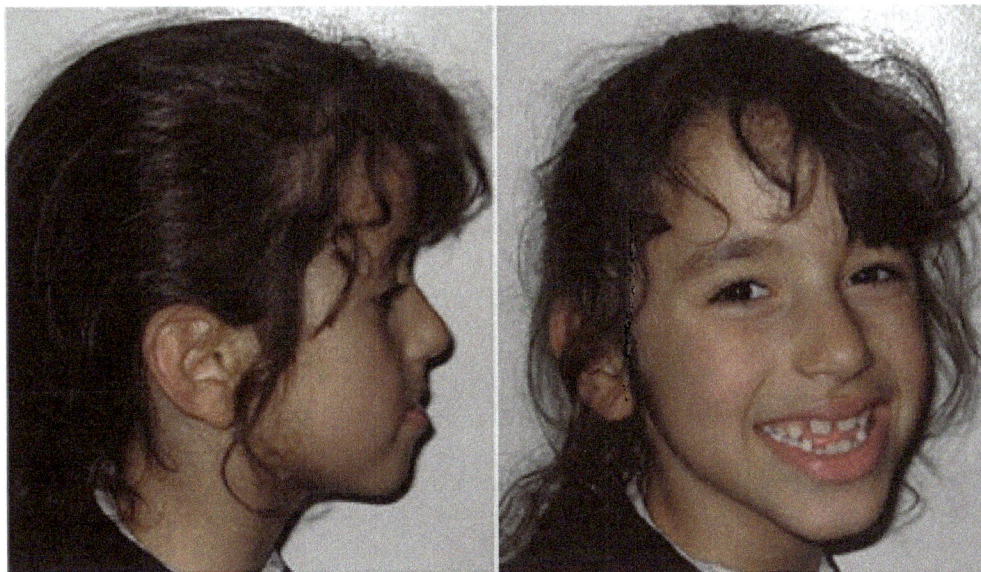

Figure 3. A patient, aged 8, presents skeletal Class III malocclusion characterized by concave profile and retrusive nasomaxillary area.

3.1.2. Endobuccal evaluation

Endobuccal exam allows the practician to identify his patient as a class I case. In skeletal Class III, dento-alveolar components compensations occur in the form of proclined maxillary incisors and retroclined mandibular incisors [9]. This is in contrast with pseudo-Class III cases, where anterior crossbite occlusion and Angle's Class III molars and canines are associated with dental compensations of class II malocclusion (Figure 4).

The assessment of dental relations must always be done with the mandible in centric relation. (Figure 5) It is important at this stage to proceed to the unique gesture, which allows making the differential diagnosis: It is the De Nevreze procedure, which consists in obtaining a more retrusive position of the mandible to minimize the dental relations in pseudo-prognathsm cases. Conversely, in true mesiocclusion, the maneuver does not succeed. The mandible cannot be retruded, and there is no modification of the dental reports [1, 15].

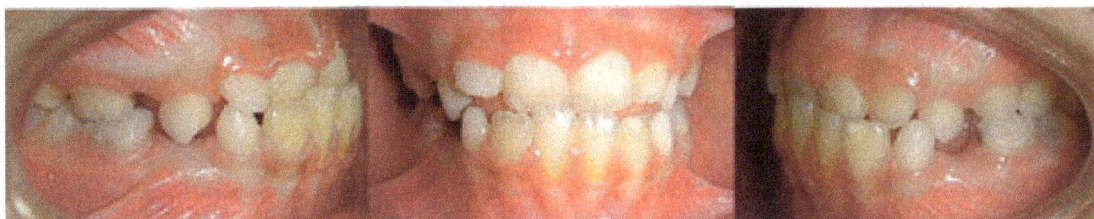

Figure 4. Pre-treatment intra-oral photographs in habitual occlusion showing characteristics of Angle's Class III molars and canines, vertical axis of the maxillary incisors, and the presence of anterior crossbite occlusion.

When the anterior crossbite exhibit a functional shift; that is, interincisal contact is possible in centric relationship, implying a pseudo Class III malocclusion with no inherent skeletal Class III discrepancy [8]. We find Characteristics of Angle's Class I molars and canines (Figure 5).

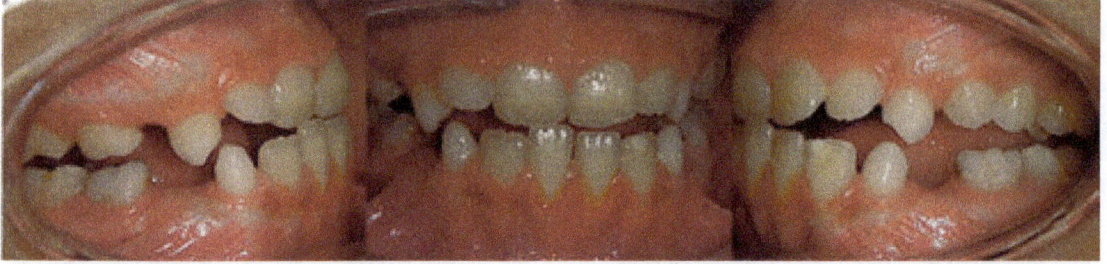

Figure 5. Pre-treatment intra-oral photographs in centric occlusion showing edge-to-edge occlusion and Angle's Class I molars and canines relationship.

3.2. Radiographic analysis

Lateral cephalogram largely contributes to establishing the diagnostic of a skeletal Class I. To evaluate the amount of mandibular shift, two lateral cephalograms, one at maximum intercuspation and one at the point of initial contact, are compared. (Figures 6)

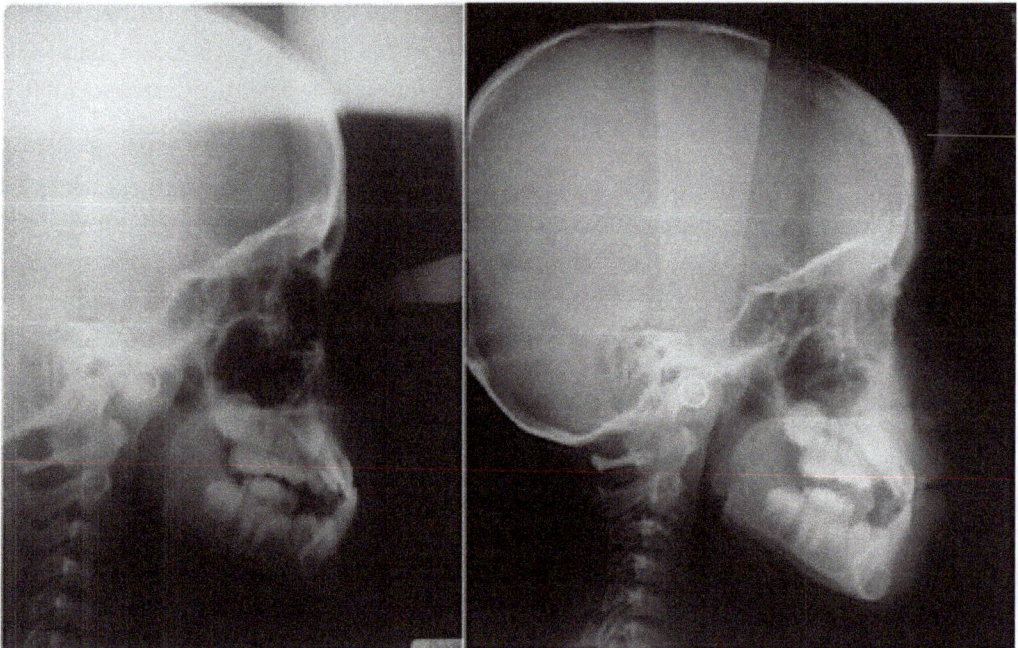

Figure 6. Pretreatment lateral cephalogram in maximum intercuspation position (AOBO=-7mm) and in position of initial contact with anterior edge to edge (AOBO=-4mm), showing that cephalometric values are in favor of a middle Class I.

In true Class III, the skeletal components are characterized by an underdeveloped maxilla, overdeveloped mandible or a combination of both. Dento-alveolar compensations are revealed by cephalometric values for proclined maxillary incisors and retroclined mandibular incisors.

Tweed defined a pseudo Class III malocclusion as having a conventionally shaped mandible. The sagittal jaw relation's show a Class I or a mild Class III pattern in centric relation. The upper incisors are often retroclined, whereas lower incisors are normally inclined or proclined [9].

4. Interceptive treatment

4.1. Timing

Optimum treatment timing for orthodontic problems continues to be one of the most controversial topics in orthodontics; this is especially true for the correction of Class III malocclusion [16].

However, spontaneous worsening during transition from deciduous to permanent dentition has been reported. For this reason, pseudo Class III malocclusion should be treated as early as possible to reduce the functional shift of the mandible and increase maxillary arch length [3, 5].

Several clinicians believe that early intervention has many advantages; they have suggested a number of reasons for early correction of anterior crossbite even in the deciduous dentition. The optimum period suggested for treatment is between 6 years and 9 years; intervention at this period permits normal growth [10].

4.2. Objectives

Generally, interceptive orthodontic treatment during mixed dentition is more effective to improve malocclusions than no treatment. Early intervention is, therefore, recommended preventing adverse effects on growth and development of the jaws and disturbance of temporal and masseter muscle activity, which would increase the risk of craniomandibular disorders during adolescence. A pseudo Class III malocclusion should be treated as early as possible to reduce the functional shift of the mandible and increase maxillary arch length [2, 3, 5].

In addition to its effectiveness and efficiency, early orthodontic treatment may have positive effects on the quality of life for both children and their families (self-esteem, social acceptance) [3].

The management of a pseudo-class III malocclusion via the proclination of upper incisors and/ or retroclination of lower incisors aims to correct anterior crossbite and eliminate mandibular displacement. Obtaining a front stop to lock the occlusion allows creating conditions for normal occlusal development [4, 9].

4.3. Modalities of treatment

Various appliances have been devised for early treatment of a pseudo Class III ; these include removable plates, fixed or removable inclined planes, functional appliances, face mask, and simple fixed appliances. Each device has its specific indication, its advantages and disadvantages [6, 10, 15].

4.3.1. Removable appliances

Hawley appliance with auxiliary springs is one of the earliest appliances introduced to produce proclination of upper incisors. The plate stabilization is provided by Adams clasp and the heightening of occlusion is strongly required to resolve an anterior crossbite (Figure 7 and 8).

A modified Hawley appliance with inverted labial bow is a simple way to manage pseudo Class III. The appliance is easy to construct and require trasferring the bite by guiding the mandible distally in an edge to edge (Figure 9) [15].

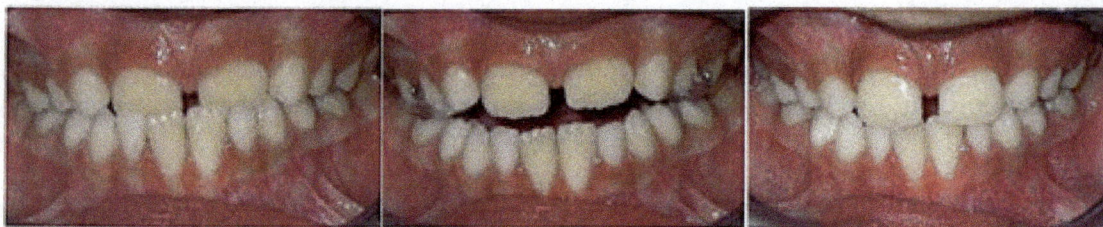

Figure 7. Correction of anterior crossbite by Hawley appliance with auxiliary springs

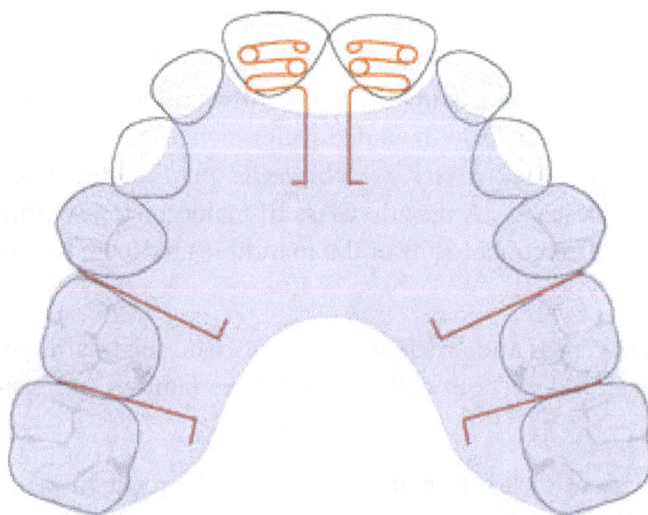

Figure 8. illustrating components of Hawley appliance with springs.

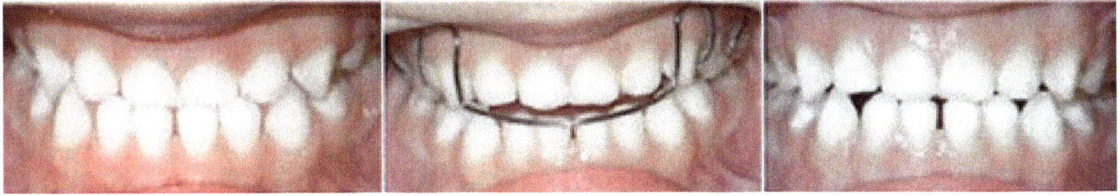

Figure 9. Correction of anterior crossbite, in deciduous dentition, by Hawley appliance with inverted labial bow

4.3.2. A modified quad helix appliance

This is one of the earliest appliances introduced for posterior expansion, it is made of 0.036 Blue Elgiloy and soldered to the bands on the first permanent maxillary molars. It can be modified by addition of an anterior extension arm. The appliance is expanded and cemented. The occlusion must be relieved by posterior bite-blocks to permit crossbite correction [9]. The gradually activation of both arms allows proclination maxillary incisors. The major indication of such device is the combination of anterior and posterior crossbites (Figure 10).

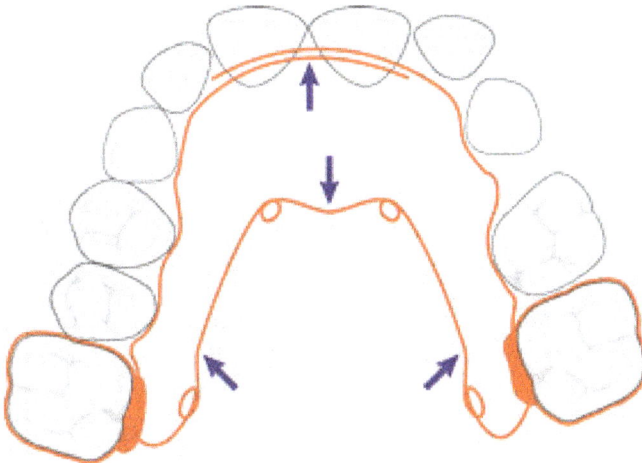

Figure 10. Illustrating activation of modified quad helix

4.3.3. Inclined plane

Some modalities for anterior crossbite correction include fixed or removable acrylic inclined planes (Croll, 1984), bonded resin-composite slopes (Bayrak and Tunc, 2008) [4, 12].

These are simple functional appliances placed on the lower arch; they allow quicker results. One of the identified advantages of removable appliance is that it can also be used as retention appliance after active treatment as well as it is possible to add acrylic teeth if necessary (Figure 11) [12].

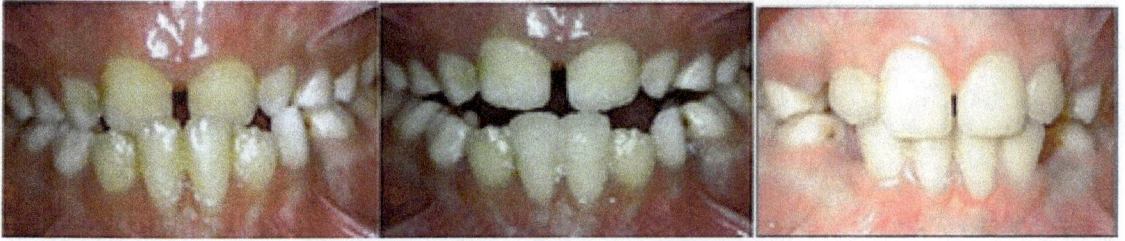

Figure 11. Correction of anterior crossbite by bonded resin-composite plane on mandibular incisors. The ramps should be progressively reduced.

4.3.4. Fixed appliance

The earlier treatment of pseudo-prognathism was feasible from a simple fixed appliance (partial bonding of brackets) simultaneously with elastics.

The most common pattern is to bond the brackets on the labial surfaces of the lower incisors and the palatal surfaces of the upper incisors. Intermaxillary elastics are then used to create an earlier proclination maxillary incisors and retroclination mandibular incisors.

This can also be composed of bands or tubes on the first permanent maxillary molars, brackets on the maxillary, and a wire with open coil springs. Brackets are also bonded on the mandibular incisors and the anterior cross-bite is simultaneously managed with Class III elastics (Figure 12) [17].

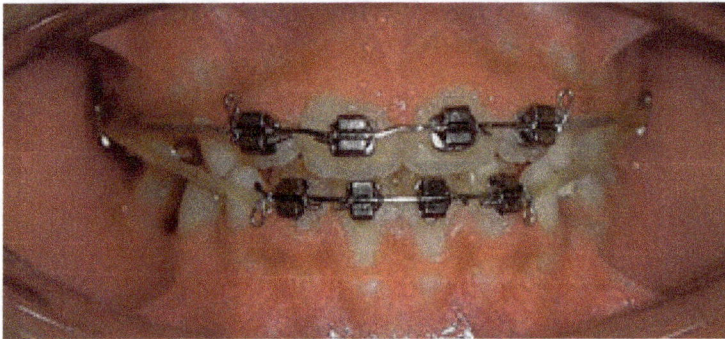

Figure 12. The components of standard edgewise appliance to resolve an anterior crossbite.

5. Case reports

5.1. Case N° 1

A 8 year-old girl was referred by her pediatric dentist for an orthodontic consultation regarding her anterior bite. Extra orally, she had a balanced face, *a slight retrusion of the upper lip while excessive mandibular anterior displacement is revealed to smile view. She presented in the early mixed dentition stage with* Class III left molar relationships. The anterior crossbite was expressed as a result of functional shift of the mandible in the sagittal plane due to lingually-inclined maxillary incisors and supernumerary anterior teeth in mandible. (Figure 13) When the mandible is manipulated into a terminal hinge-axis position, the incisors come into edge-to-edge contact, requiring the patient to move the mandible forward to achieve posterior occlusion. The panoramic radiograph showed presumptive signs of crowding in the maxilla. The cephalometric values confirmed retroclined maxillary incisors, proclined mandibular incisors, and normal vertical development. (Figure 14)

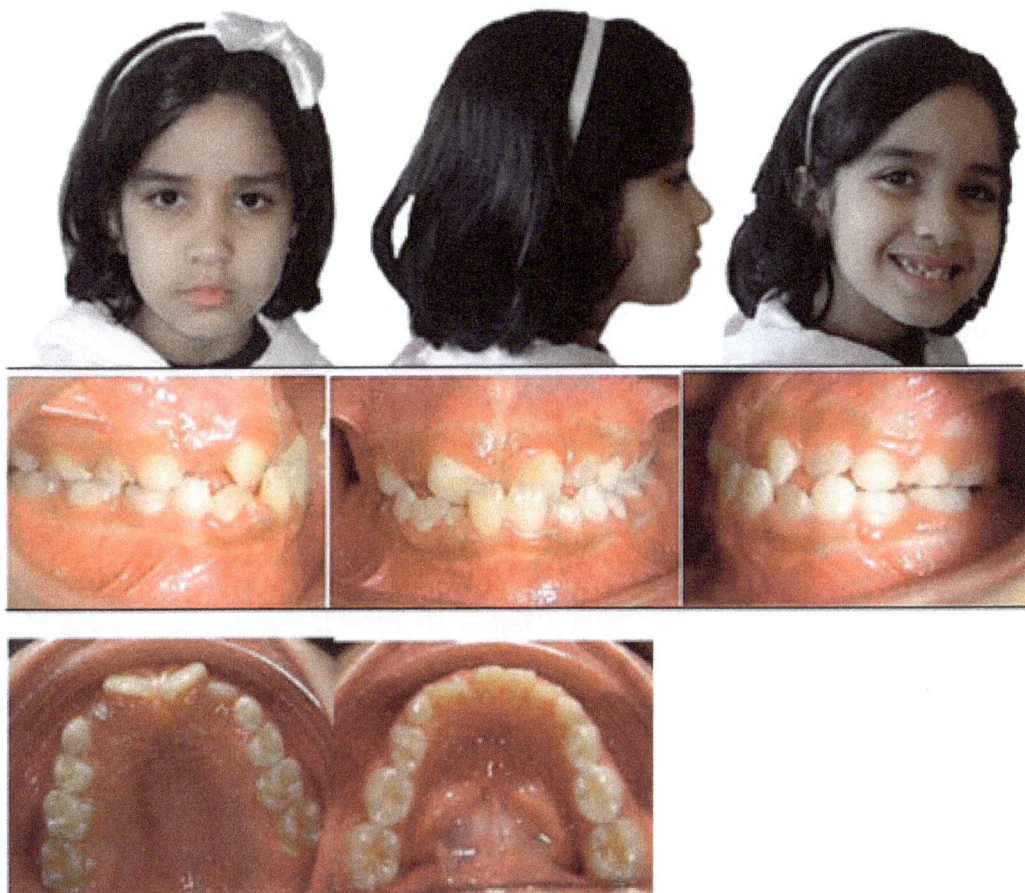

Figure 13. Pre-treatment extraoral and intraoral photographs.

The treatment aims to reduce the functional shift of the mandible and increase maxillary arch length, thus permitting eruption of the permanent canines and premolars into a Class I relationship. Bonding brackets to the two maxillary permanent central incisors in combination with banding the two maxillary permanent first molars was used. The device consists, in the first stage, of a round stainless steel arch wire to achieve alignment of upper incisors; an elevation of the occlusion was provided by resin-composite bite plane bonded to lingual side of the lower incisors. Then, an open-coil spring was compressed against the molar tube to push the incisors labially. So, the supernumerary incisor was extracted for the recovery of the lower incisor. (Figure 15)

The total active treatment period was about 6 months and follow-up appointments were scheduled every 4 weeks. Upon completion of treatment, the anterior crossbite was corrected, the molar relationships were restored to Class I. Advancing the maxillary incisors labially normalized the overjet and allow the mandible to close into a Class I without the anterior shift. Finally the treatment improved maxillary lip posture and facial appearance (Figure 16) Both skeletal and dento-alveolar effects of interceptive treatment are illustrated in Figure 15; the wits appraisal is a leading indicator of re-equilibration of maxillomandibular relationship (AOBO=0mm). (Figure 17)

The case was followed up out of retention 6 months later. Stable anterior and posterior relationships were evident, and continued spontaneous alignment of the mandibular incisors was noticed. (Figure 18)

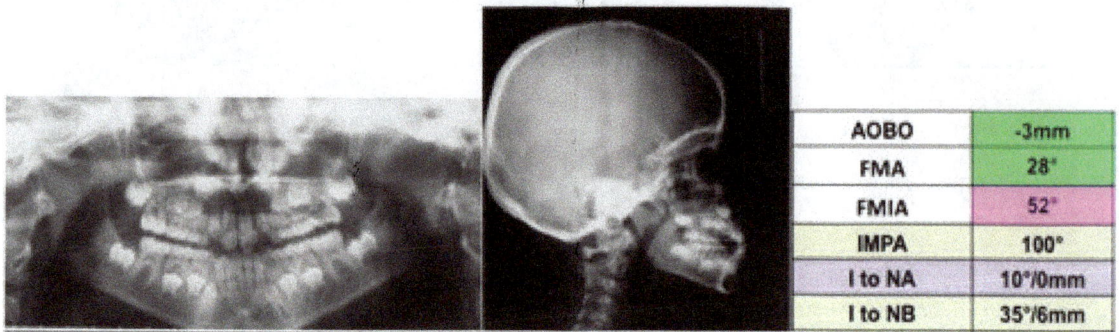

AOBO	-3mm
FMA	28°
FMIA	52°
IMPA	100°
I to NA	10°/0mm
I to NB	35°/6mm

Figure 14. Pre-treatment radiographs.

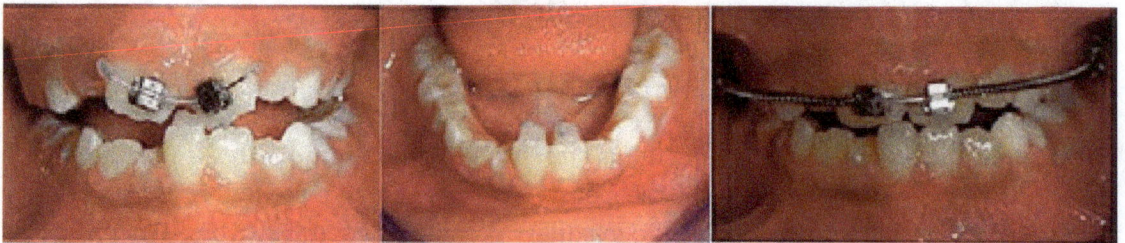

Figure 15. Treatment progress.

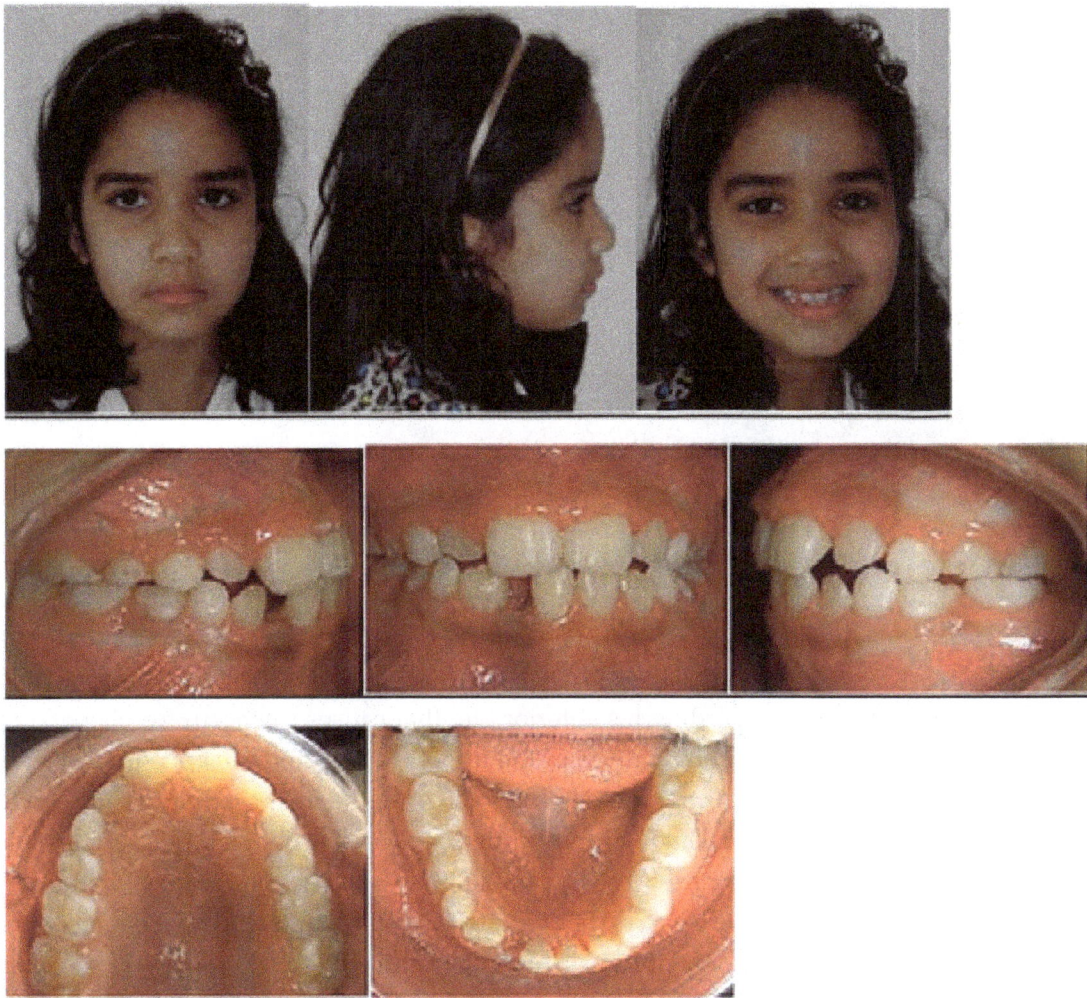

Figure 16. Extraoral and intraoral photographs after anterior crossbite correction.

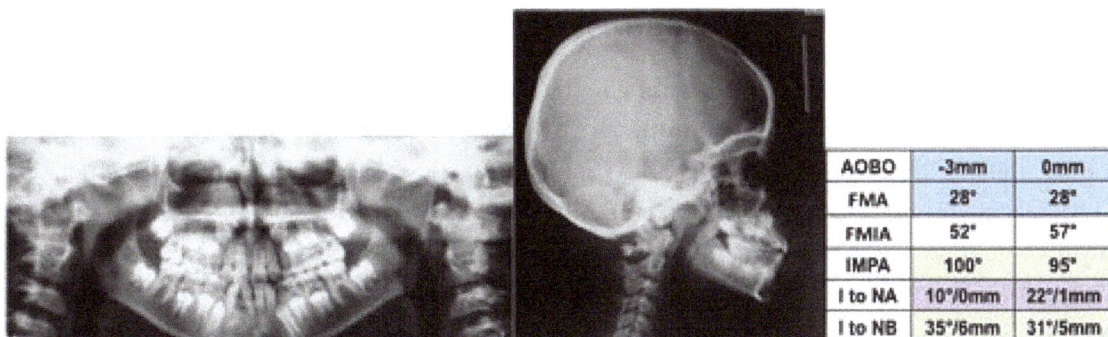

AOBO	-3mm	0mm
FMA	28°	28°
FMIA	52°	57°
IMPA	100°	95°
I to NA	10°/0mm	22°/1mm
I to NB	35°/6mm	31°/5mm

Figure 17. post-treatment radiographs.

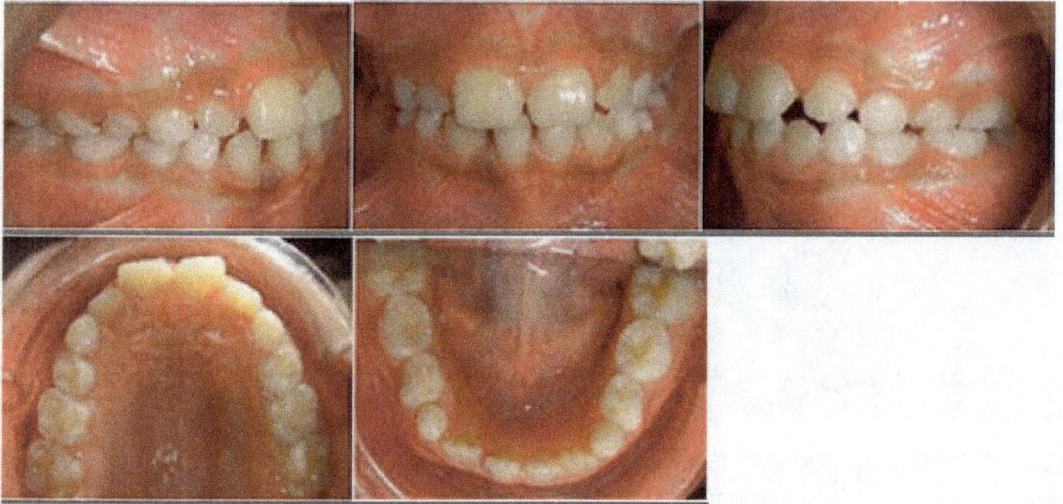

Figure 18. Six months post-treatment intraoral photographs.

5.2. Case N° 2

A 9-year-old boy consulted regarding his anterior bite that causes a concern for his parents. On extraoral examination, a slight retrusion of the upper lip was noticed, and smile betrays the anterior reversed occlusion. Intraoral examination revealed a mixed dentition stage, with erupted upper and lower permanent incisors and first molars. All maxillary incisors were in crossbite with the mandibular incisors. The molar relation on both sides was developing class III malocclusion (Figure 19). There was no family history of class III malocclusion. On assessment guidance of the mandible on closure, a functional shift of the mandible was seen. An occlusal prematurity in relation to erupting 41 and retroclination of maxillary incisors appeared to be responsible for the present functional shift [Figure 20]. Based on the above findings, a diagnosis of pseudo class III malocclusion was made and the treatment aimed at eliminating the anterior interlock. It was expected to position the mandible backward and promote maxillary growth with standard edgewise appliance.

Bite opening and bracket and tube bonding to the four maxillary incisors and the two maxillary permanent first molars (2 * 4 fixed appliance) were used to resolve an anterior crossbite in combination with open coil spring and Class III elastics (Figure 21). After leveling and alignment stage, crossbite was corrected in 4 months. After six months of treatment, significant improvement in the patient's profile and smile was noted. An increase in upper incisor inclination was obtained, and reduction in lower incisor inclination resulted in normalized overbite and overjet. So, for more security, we opted for a bonded maxillary retainer (Figure 22). The effects observed were attributed to the correction of interlocking and also to the guidance of the mandible in a normal backward position. The intraoral examination after a 1-year follow-up revealed a normal overjet and overbite relation [Figure 23].

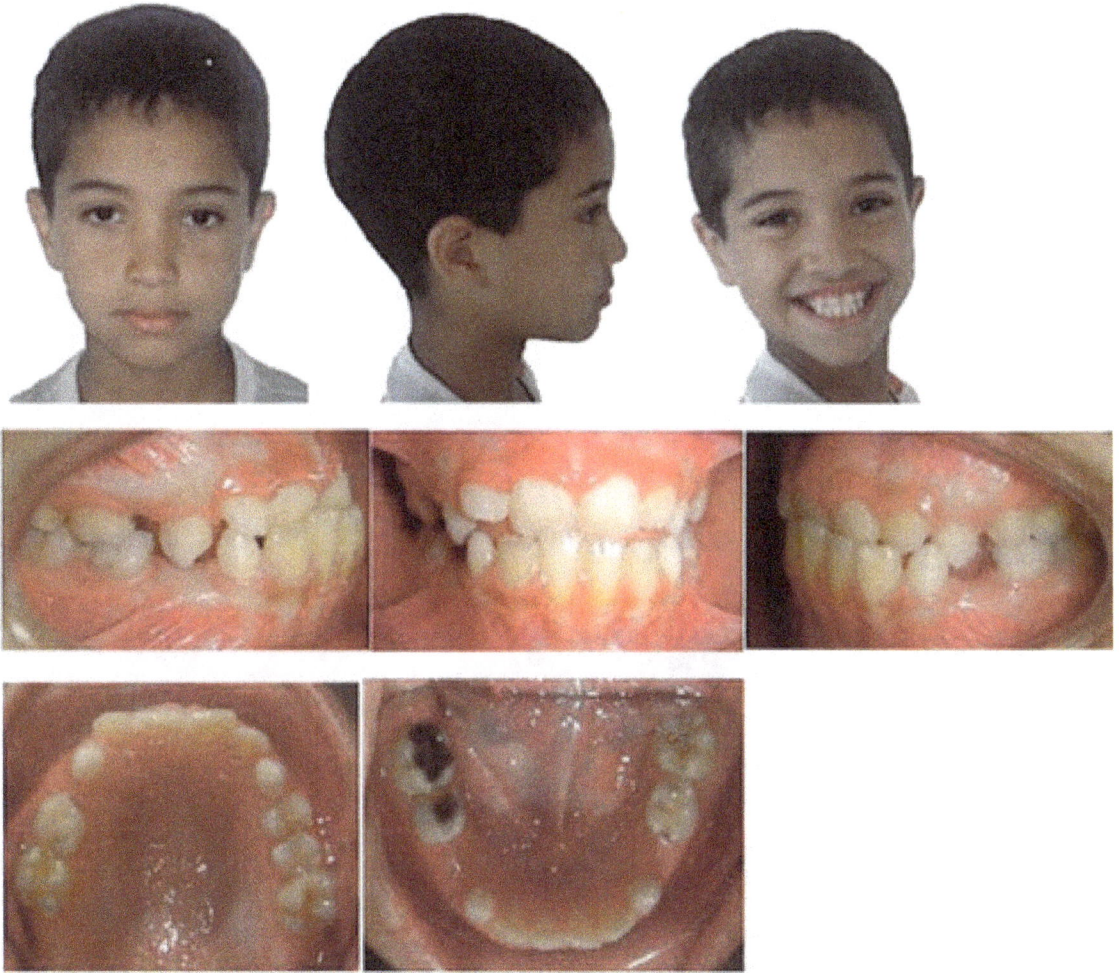

Figure 19. Pre-treatment extraoral and intraoral photographs.

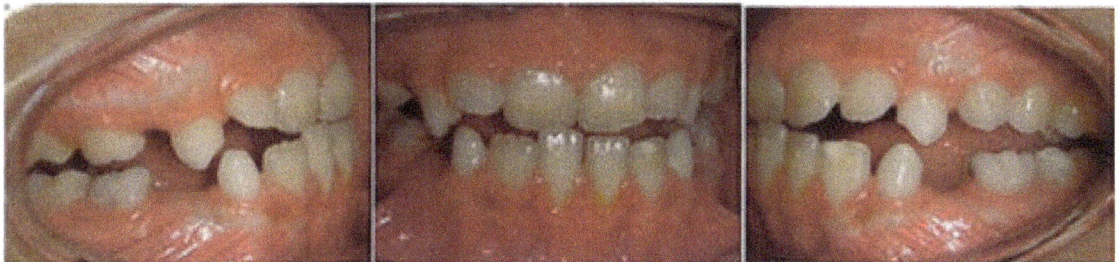

Figure 20. Pre-treatment intra-oral photographs in centric occlusion.

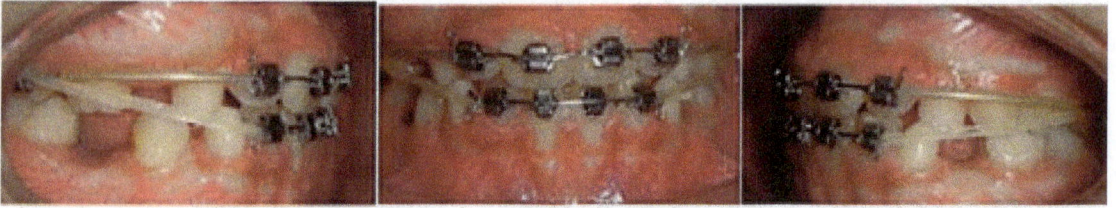

Figure 21. Upper and lower 2*4 appliances in combination with Class III elastics, used for advancing maxillary incisors into desired overjet.

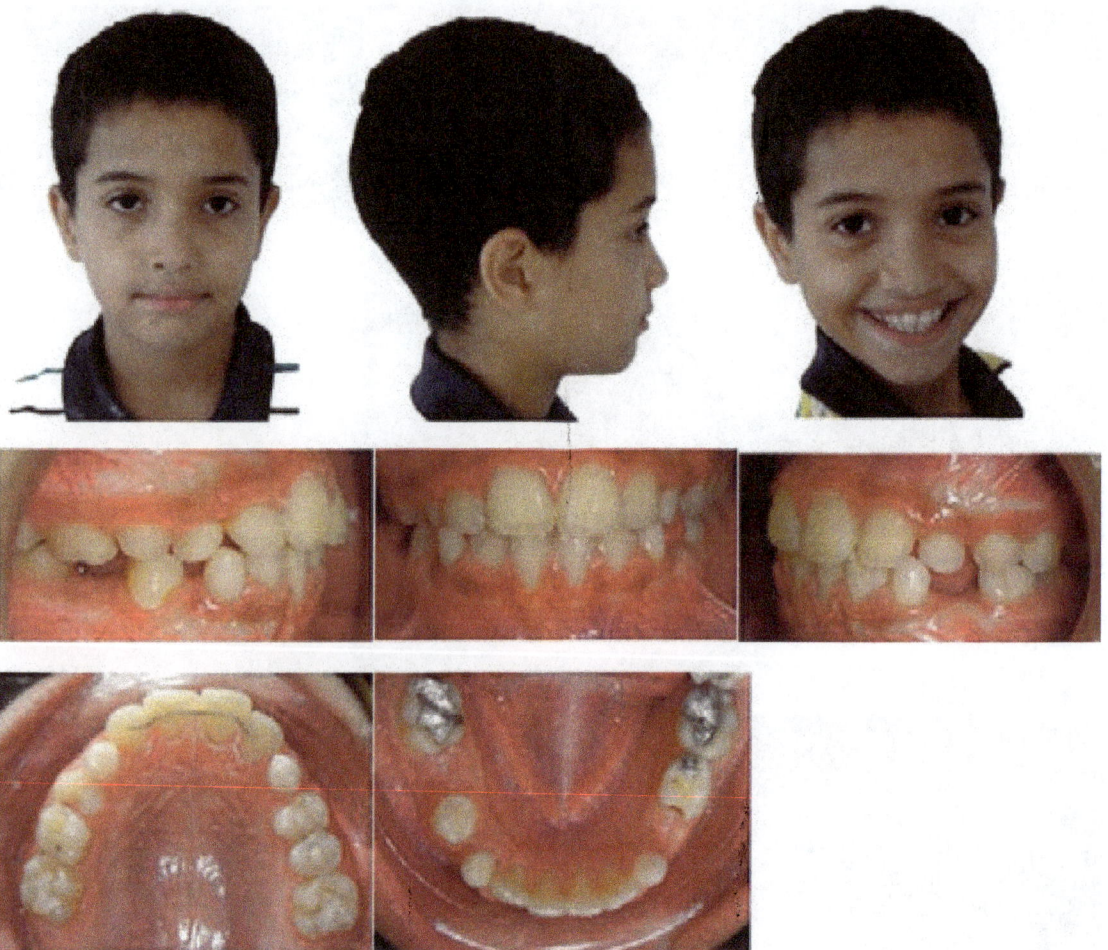

Figure 22. Extraoral and intraoral photographs after anterior crossbite correction.

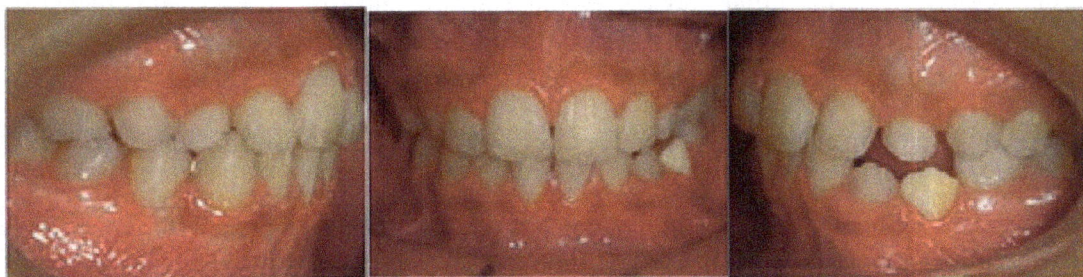

Figure 23. Year-follow-up

6. Discussion

Anterior crossbite is a major concern for both parents and clinicians. It requires early intervention to achieve a normal occlusion that is morphologically stable in the long term and functionally and esthetically acceptable. However the fundamental goal of interceptive approach is to improve the growth.

The pseudo-Class III malocclusion involves both permanent teeth and deciduous dentition. Some practitioners prefer to wait for the permanent maxillary incisors to erupt before initiating therapy due to the natural tendency of teeth to erupt in a lingual position during dental arch development. And the possible spontaneous correction of functional deciduous anterior crossbites occasionally corrects themselves spontaneously. However, the optimum period for successful treatment suggested being between the ages 6–9 years [10].

Interceptive orthodontic procedures must be relatively simple and inexpensive treatment approaches that target developing malocclusions during the mixed dentition. In cases of pseudo-Class III malocclusion, early intervention has a highly favorable cost-benefit ratio, and treatment usually takes less time [18]. So, it was suggested that early management of anterior crossbite in these kind of case be successful in 100% of treated young patients [17].

The various treatments suggested in the literature for correction of anterior crossbite include different appliances, both fixed and/or removable with heavy intermittent forces (inclined bite plane, tongue blade) or light-continuous forces (removable appliance with auxiliary springs). A recent systematic review disclosed a wide variety of treatment modalities, more than 12 methods, in use for anterior crossbite correction [19]. However, strong evidence in support of any treatment technique is lacking [8].

Removable appliances have been shown to be effective in the correction of anterior crossbite and elimination of mandibular displacement. Nonetheless, the major inconvenience of these tools is the necessity of an absolute cooperation on the part of the patient due to a high risk of loss or repetitive fractures.

A modified quad helix appliance has proved to be an economical alternative, which is easy to fabricate and causes minimal patient discomfort [9].

Other alternative therapies that may correct skeletal problems in young patients have been shown to be effective in functional Class III, with significant changes in the craniofacial complex, including the use of protraction headgear, chin cup, and Frankel III [10, 15].

The face mask should be advised during the deciduous dentition phase in cases of minor skeletal component. This produces protrusive forces to the maxilla and maxillary dentition.

The literature demonstrates that functional appliances are effective in anterior crossbite correction. This approach prevents unfavourable growth especially mandibular protrusion, and eliminates traumatic occlusion. Giancotti suggested the therapeutic use of a Balters' Bionator appliance. The patients wore the bionator approximately 15 hours daily for a period of 60-90 days. However, the cooperation of the patient is essential for the success of this approach [10].

Bonding brackets to the four maxillary incisors in combination with banding or bonding the two maxillary permanent first molars is one of the methods used for the correction of anterior crossbite with fixed appliances. It has been reported to effectively manage anterior crossbite in the mixed dentition [20]. For some authors, the main reason for using the fixed appliance treatment seems to be misalignment, [17] For others, this method has the advantages of requiring little or no patient compliance or alteration of speech [4].

One of the benefits claimed for early treatment with fixed appliance is that space is provided for the eruption of the canines and premolars in the upper arch, allowing the erupting dentition to be guided into a Class I relationship in centric relation [17].

There is disagreement about the need for a second phase of treatment during adolescence, A retrospective cohort study of interceptive orthodontic treatment indicate that interceptive orthodontic treatment is effective for improving malocclusion, but does not produce finished-quality results without a second phase of treatment in the permanent dentition [3]. Several studies have suggested that systematically planned interceptive treatment in the mixed dentition might contribute to a significant reduction in treatment need between the ages of 8 and 12 years, In a Finnish study, the need was reduced significantly from 8 to 12. However, Only 25% of these patients required a second stage of treatment after eruption of the remaining permanent teeth [21].

With respect to stability of such approach, it was reported, in follow-up study, that in young patients diagnosed with pseudo Class III malocclusion and treated early with a fixed appliance, the overjet was corrected, and the treatment result was maintained in the long term (for mor than 5 years after active treatment) [17]. So, it was suggested that either fixed or removable appliances with similar long-term stability could successfully correct anterior crossbite [22].

A systematic review of early correction of anterior crossbite has highlighted the lack of high quality evidence, and concludes that despite the low level of evidence, there is similarity in the length of time it took to successfully treat anterior crossbites using similar treatment modalities [19].

The therapeutic use of a fixed appliance is suggested in two case reports of subjects with anterior crossbite in mixed dentition. Careful clinical evaluation of Class III malocclusion checked anterior and posterior dental relationships with the mandible in centric relation. The prognosis was favorable for the treatment and post-retention results to be stable in the future. The two patients achieved a positive and often slightly overcorrected overjet during the active treatment after six months of treatment.

As early correction of anterior crossbite was undertaken in the growing child, it is important to evaluate post-treatment changes. The overjet remained stable because the corrected upper incisors were kept in place by normalizing the overjet and overbite.

7. Conclusion

Interceptive orthodontic treatment aims to recognize and eliminate potential irregularities and malpositions in the developing dento-facial complex. Early treatment of Class III malocclusion is one of the most challenging problems confronting orthodontists. The treatment should be carried out as early as possible with the aim of permitting normal growth, and improving facial attractiveness and psychosocial well being of children.

In spite of its weak prevalence, functional Class III must be prematurely detected and treated to prevent a functional anomaly from becoming a skeletal anomaly. A well-conducted clinical and radiographic examination, highlighting skeletal Class I, allows judicious and appropriate therapeutic choices.

The optimum treatment timing and the treatment modalities influence therapy. It is believed to have many benefits, including a better use of the patient's growth potential, a lower risk of progression to a true Class III malocclusion, and more stable results.

Author details

Sanaa Alami[1*], Hakima Aghoutan[1], Farid El Quars[1], Samir Diouny[2] and Farid Bourzgui[1]

*Address all correspondence to: alamisana89@gmail.com

1 Department of Dento-facial Orthopedic, Faculty of Dental Medicine, Hassan II University of Casablanca, Morocco

2 Chouaib Doukkali University, Faculty of Letters & Human Sciences, El Jadida, Morocco

References

[1] Le Gall M, Philip C, Bandon D. The functional mandibular prognathism. Archives de pédiatrie. 2009; 16; 77–83.

[2]   Keski-Nisula K, Lehto R, Lusa V, Keski-Nisula L, Varrela J. Occurrence of malocclu-sion and need of orthodontic treatment in early mixed dentition. Am J Orthod Dento-facial Orthop. 2003; 124:631-8.

[3]   King GJ, Brudvik P. Effectiveness of interceptive orthodontic treatment in reducing malocclusions. Am J Orthod Dentofacial Orthop. 2010;137;18-25.

[4]   Bindayel NA. Simple removable appliances to correct anterior and posterior cross-bite in mixed dentition: Case report. The Saudi Dental Journal. 2012; 24, 105–13.

[5]   Kumar A, Tandon P, Singh GP. Management of pseudo Class III malocclusion-syner-gistic approach with fixed and functional appliance. Int J Orthod Milwaukee. 2013; 24 (2) 41-4.

[6]   Randrianarimanarivo HM, Rasoanirina MO, Andriambololo-Nivo RD, Ralison G, Ra-kotovao JD. Interception de la pseudo-prognathie mandibulaire: comparaison de la plaque en "V" et du plan incliné antéro-inférieur. Revue d'odontostomatologie malg-ache en ligne. 2011; 3; 29-38.

[7]   Langlade M. Diagnostic orthodontique, Paris : Maloine ;1981.

[8]   Wiedel AP, Bondemark L. Stability of anterior crossbite correction: A randomized controlled trial with a 2-year follow-up. Angle Orthod. 2014.

[9]   Kumar A, SA, Shetty KS, Prakash AT. Pseudo-Class III: Diagnosis and Simplistic Treatment. J Ind Orthod Soc. 2011; 45 (4) 198-201.

[10] Giancotti A, Maselli A, Mampieri G, Spanò E. Pseudo-Class III malocclusion treat-ment with Balters' Bionator. Journal of Orthodontics. 2003; 30; 203–15.

[11] Ngan P1, Hu AM, Fields HW Jr. Treatment of Class III problems begins with differ-ential diagnosis of anterior crossbites. Pediatr Dent. 1997 Sep-Oct;19(6):386-95.

[12] Jirgensone I, Liepa A, Abeltins A. Anterior crossbite correction in primary and mixed dentition with removable inclined plane (Bruckl appliance). Stomatologija. 2008;10 (4):140-4.

[13] Park JH. Orthodontic correction of Class III malocclusion in a young patient with the use of a simple fixed appliance. Int J Orthod Milwaukee. 2012 ; 23 (3 43-8.

[14] Arman A, Ufuk Toygar T, Abuhijleh E. Profile Changes Associated with Different Orthopedic Treatment Approaches in Class III Malocclusions Angle Orthodontist. 2004; 74 (6) 733-40.

[15] Negi KS, Sharma KR. Treatment of pseudo Class III malocclusion by modified Haw-leys appliance with inverted labial bow. Journal of Indian Society of Pedodontics and Preventive Dentistry. 2011; 29 (1) 57-61.

[16] Le Gall M, Philip C, Salvadori A. Early treatment of Class III malocclusion. Orthod Fr. 2011;82 (3) 241-52.

[17] Hägg U, DDS, Tse A, Bendeus M, Rabie ABM. A Follow-up Study of Early Treatment of Pseudo Class III Malocclusion. Angle Orthodontist, Vol 74, No 4, 2004.

[18] Bowman SJ. A Quick Fix for Pseudo-Class III Correction. J. clin Ortho. 2008; 42(10) 1-7.

[19] Borrie F1, Bearn D. Early correction of anterior crossbites: a systematic review. J Orthod. 2011; 38(3) 175-84.

[20] Dowsing P1, Sandler PJ. How to effectively use a 2 x 4 appliance. J Orthod. 2004; 31(3) 248-58.

[21] Gu, Y.; Rabie, A.B.; and Hägg, U.Treatment effects of simple fixed appliance and reverse headgear in correction of anterior crossbites, Am. J. Orthod. 2000.117:691-99,

[22] Wiedel AP, Bondemark L. Stability of anterior crossbite correction: A randomized controlled trial with a 2-year follow-up. Angle Orthodontist. 2014.

2

Interceptive Orthodontics — Current Evidence

Maen H. Zreaqat

1. Introduction

From evidence found in human skulls, crooked teeth have been around since the time of Neanderthal man (about 50,000 BC), but it was not until about 3000 years ago that we had the first written record of attempts to correct crowded or protruding teeth. Long before braces, long before the word orthodontics" was coined, it was known that teeth moved in response to pressure. Primitive (and surprisingly well-designed) orthodontic appliances have been found with Greek and Etruscan artifacts. Archaeologists have discovered Egyptian mummies with crude metal bands wrapped around individual teeth. It is speculated that catgut was used to close the gaps [1]. The earliest description of irregularities of the teeth was given about 400 BC by Hippocrates (460-377 BC). The first treatment of an irregular tooth was recorded by Celsus (25 BC-50 AD), a Roman writer, who said, "If a second tooth should happen to grow in children before the first has fallen out, that which ought to be shed is to be drawn out and the new one daily pushed toward its place by means of the finger until it arrives at its just proportion." A clear mechanical treatment was advocated by Pliny the Elder (23-79 AD), who suggested filing elongated teeth to bring them into proper alignment. This method remained in practice until the 1800s [2].

Dentistry entered a period of marked decline during middle ages (5th to 15th centuries), as did all sciences. After the 16th century, considerable progress was made. Matthaeus Gottfried Purmann (1692) was the first to report taking wax impressions. In 1756, Phillip Pfaff used plaster of Paris impressions. Malocclusions were called "irregularities" of the teeth, and their correction was termed "regulating." It remained for the Enlightenment to reawaken the spirit of scientific thought necessary to advance dentistry and other disciplines. Beginning in the 18th century, Pierre Fauchard (1678-1761) was leading efforts in the field of dentistry. He has been called the "Father of Orthodontia." He was the first to remove dentistry from the bonds of empiricism and put it on a scientific foundation. In 1728, he published the first general work on dentistry, a 2-volume opus entitled "The Surgeon Dentist: A Treatise on the Teeth".

Fauchard described for first time the bandeau, an expansion arch consisting of a horseshoe-shaped strip of precious metal to which the teeth were ligated (Fig 1). This became the basis for Angle's E-arch, and even today its principles are used in unraveling a crowded dentition. He also "repositioned" teeth with a forceps, called a "pelican" because of its resemblance to the beak of that bird, and ligated the tooth to its neighbors until healing took place. At that time, little attention was paid to anything other than the alignment of teeth and then almost exclusively to the maxilla. moreover, he was the first to recommend serial extraction by extracting premolars to relieve crowding [3].

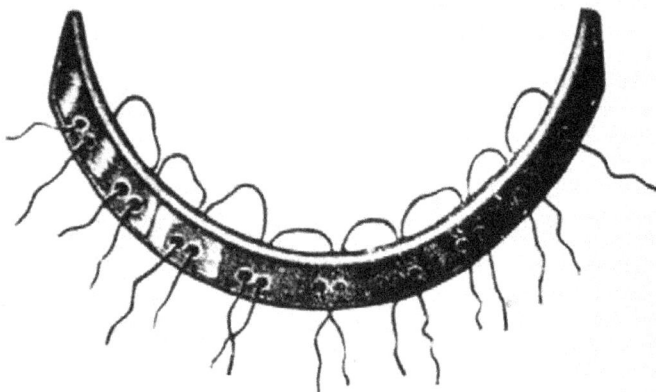

Figure 1. Fauchard's bandeau

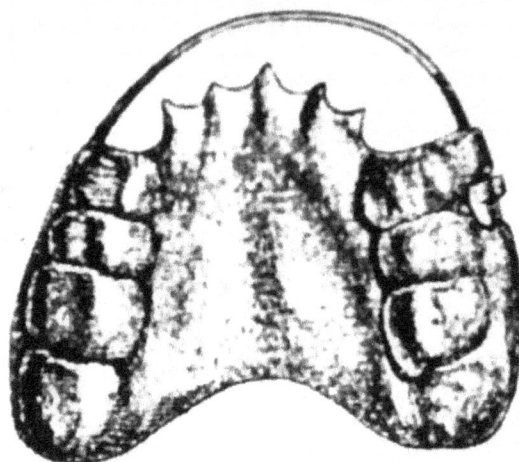

Figure 2. Removable "plate" used by Friedrich Christoph

Friedrich Christoph Kneisel (1797-1847), a German dentist, was the first to use plaster models to record malocclusion and removable appliance to fit prognathic teeth with a chin strap (Fig.

2). However, before the time of Edward Angle, the treatment of malocclusions was chaotic, with little understanding of normal occlusion and even less understanding of the development of the dentition. Appliances were primitive, not only in design but also in the metals and materials used. There was no rational basis for diagnosis and case analysis. It was Edward Hartley Angle (1855 –1930), early in the 20th century, who dominated the emergence of "orthodontia as a science and a specialty". He also created the first educational program to train specialists in orthodonticsand he developed the first prefabricated orthodontic appliance system. Angle is considered the father' of modern orthodontics [4].

2. The development of the occlusion of the teeth

The primary dentition begins to erupt at the age of about 6 months, and is normally completely in occlusion by about 3 years of age. Details of mean age of eruption and the range of variation have been reported by Van der Linden (1983) for Swedish children and by Sato and Ogiwara (1971) for Japanese children. There appear to be no significant differences between the sexes for the age of primary tooth eruption. The first teeth to erupt and to form occlusal contacts are the incisors, which ideally take up occlusal positions that are more vertical than the permanent incisors, with a deeper incisal overbite. The lower incisors in this condition will contact the cingulum area of the upper incisors in centric occlusion. Spaces are present between the primary incisor teeth. Following eruption of the incisors, the first primary molars erupt into occlusion. These teeth take up occlusal contacts so that the lower molars are slightly forward in relation to the upper molar. The last teeth to erupt into occlusion in the primary dentition are the second molars. These teeth erupt slightly spaced from the first molars, but the space quickly closes by forward movement of the second molars which take up a position so that the distal surfaces of the upper and lower second molars are in the same vertical plane in occlusion. Thus certain features of the 'ideal' occlusion of the primary dentition when fully erupted can be described as following:

1. Spacing of incisor teeth.

2. Anthropoid spaces mesial to upper canine and distal to lower canine, into which the opposing canine interdigitates.

3. Vertical position of incisor teeth, with lower incisor touching the cingulum of upper incisor.

4. The distal surfaces of the upper and lower second primary molars in the same vertical plane.

From the age of about 6 years onwards the primary dentition is replaced by the permanent dentition. The primary incisors, canines and molars are replaced by the permanent incisors, canines and premolars, and the permanent molars erupt as additional teeth. There is some difference in size between the primary teeth and the permanent teeth which directly replace them. The permanent incisors and canines are usually larger than the corresponding primary teeth, and the premolars are usually smaller than the corresponding primary molars. Studies reported by Van der Linden (1983), have shown that the overall difference in size between the two dentitions is not large, amounting on average to about 3 mm in the upper teeth and less than 1 mm in the lower teeth. There is, however, not a strong correlation between the sizes of the primary dentition and the permanent teeth. The relationship of the jaws to each other will have a large influence on the relationship of the dental arches. The relationship of the jaws to each other can also vary in all three planes of space, and variation in any plane can affect the occlusion of the teeth. The antero-posterior positional relationship of the basal parts of the upper and lower jaws to each other, with the teeth in occlusion, is known as the skeletal relationship. This is sometimes called the dental base relationship, or the skeletal pattern. A classification of the skeletal relationship is in common use, namely:

1. Skeletal Class 1—in which the jaws are in their ideal antero-posterior relationship in occlusion.

2. Skeletal Class 2—in which the lower jaw in occlusion is positioned further back in relation to the upper jaw than in skeletal Class 1.

3. Skeletal Class 3—in which the lower jaw in occlusion is positioned further forward than in skeletal Class 1.

In addition, the teeth erupt into an environment of functional activity governed by the muscles of mastication, of the tongue and of the face. The muscles of the tongue, lips and cheeks are of particular importance in guiding the teeth into their final position, and variation in muscle form and function can affect the position and occlusion of the teeth. Moreover, some dental and local factors can affect the development of occlusion. These include: alterations in size of the dentition in relation to jaw size, crossbite, aberrant developmental position of individual teeth, presence of supernumerary teeth, developmental hypodontia, labial frenum, thumb or finger sucking. Early interference and modification of these basic etiological features can help to avoid malocclusion or reduce the need for treatment in some cases. Consequently interceptive orthodontic treatment has been set as an important aspect of orthodontic care [5].

3. Interceptive orthodontics: Definition of the concept

The concept and the necessity of interceptive orthodontic treatment, so called early, have been controversial. Some define it as removable or fixed appliance intervention in the deciduous, early mixed, or midmixed dentition. Others place it in the late mixed dentition stage of development (before emergence of the second premolars and the permanent maxillary canines). The American Association of Orthodontists' Council of Orthodontic Education defines interceptive orthodontics as "that phase of the science and art of orthodontics employed to recognize and eliminate potential irregularities and malpositions in the developing dentofacial complex." [6]. While some profession's leaders advocate that early treatment is always desirable because tissue tolerance and their power of adjustment are at or near their maximum, others warn that there is no assurance that the results of early treatment will be sustained, and that several-phased treatment will always lengthen overall treatment time.

Early treatment not only may do some damage or prolong therapy, it may exhaust the child's spirit of cooperation and compliance [7]. Joseph Fox (1776-1816, English), in his "Natural History of the Human Teeth" (London, 1803), recommended that treatment be started "before 13 or 14 years of age, and as much earlier as possible." Angle advocated the institution of orthodontic treatment "as near the beginning of the variation from the normal in the process of the development of the dental apparatus as possible". Although Nance advocated that "active treatment in the mixed dentition period is desirable only in Class III cases, crossbites, and Class II cases wherein facial appearance is markedly affected," he freed orthodontists from their hesitancy to treat patients before the development of the adult dentition [8].

4. Orthodontic interceptive measures during primary and mixed dentition

4.1. Space maintainers

The primary dentition plays a very important role in the child's growth and development, not only in terms of speech, chewing, appearance and the prevention of bad habits but also in the guidance and eruption of permanent teeth. Exfoliation of primary teeth and eruption of permanent teeth is a normal physiological process. When this normal process is disrupted, due to factors like premature loss of primary teeth, proximal carious lesions etc, it may lead to mesial migration of teeth resulting in loss of the arch length which may manifest as malocclusion in permanent dentition in the form of crowding, impaction of permanent teeth, supraeruption of opposing teeth etc. The best way to avoid these problems is to preserve the primary teeth in the arch till their normal time of exfoliation is attained. Hence it is rightly quoted that primary teeth serve as best space maintainers for permanent dentition. However, if premature extraction or loss of tooth is unavoidable due to extensive caries or other reasons, the safest option to maintain arch space is by placing a space maintainer. The fixed space maintainers are usually indicated to maintain the space created by unilateral/bilateral prema-ture loss of primary teeth in either of the arches. Of the various fixed space maintainers, Band and Loop type of space maintainers are one of the most frequently used appliances with good high success rates [9]. Cemented lower lingual bars, transpalatal arches, crowns with distal extensions are other forms of space maintainers utilizing similar mechanisms (Fig. 3) Never-theless, disintegration of cement, solder failure, caries formation along the margins of the band and long construction time are some of the disadvantages associated with them [10].

Considering this, there has been many pilot studies that explain the use of newer adhesive directly bonded splints. They are glass fiber reinforced composite resins (e.g. Ribbond, Everstick) as fixed space maintainers [11, 12]. Ribbond is a biocompatible esthetic material made from high strength polyethylene fibers (Fig. 4). The various advantages of this material includes its ease of adhesion to the dental contours, fast technique of application and good strength, well tolerated by the patient [13]. However there is limited literature is available in terms of efficacy and longevity [14].

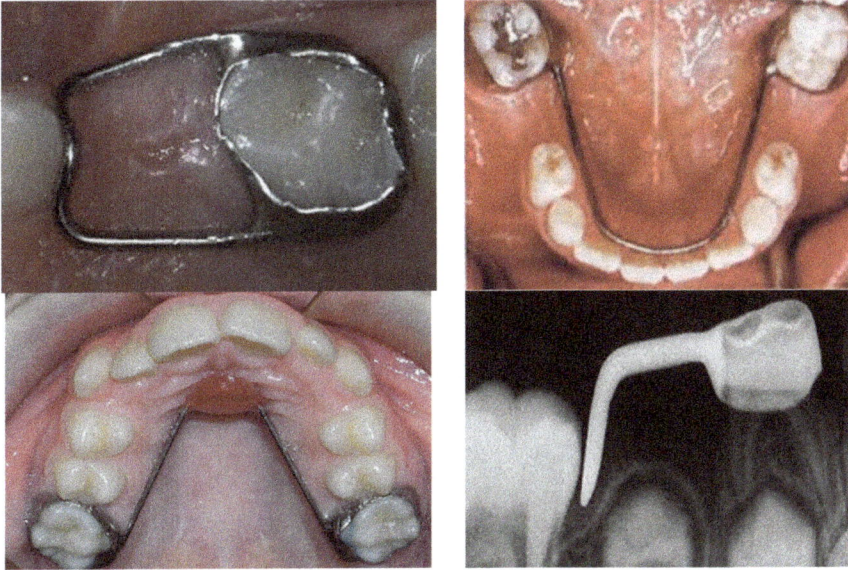

Figure 3. Various space maintainers

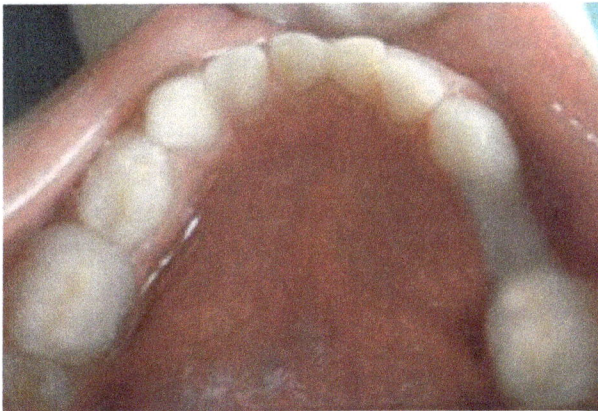

Figure 4. Ribbond space maintainer

5. Elimination of oral habits

Oral habits are learned patterns of muscle contraction and have a very complex nature. They are associated with anger, hunger, sleep, tooth eruption and fear. Some children even display oral habits for release of mental tension. These habits might be non-nutritive sucking (thumb, finger, pacifier and/or tongue), lip biting and bruxism events. These habits can result in damage to dentoalveolar structure; hence, dentists play a crucial role in giving necessary information to parents. This information includes relevant changes in the dentoalveolar structure and the method to stop oral habits. Also, a dentist is required to treat the ensuring malocclusion. The prevalence of oral habits in high school girls and primary school students has been reported to be 87.9 and 30%, respectively [15].

Oral habits could be divided into 2 main groups:

1. Acquired oral habits: Include those behaviors which are learned and could be stopped easily and when the child grows up, he or she can give up that behavior and start another one.

2. Compulsive oral habits: Consist of those behaviors which are fixed in child and when emotional pressures are intolerable for the child, he or she can feel safety with this habit, and preventing the child from these habits make him or her anxious and worried.

5.1. Thumb sucking

Thumb sucking is the most common oral habit and it is reported that its prevalence is between 13 to 60% in some societies [16]. Basically, sucking is one of an infant's natural reflexes. They begin to suck on their thumbs or other fingers while they are in the womb. Infants and young children may suck on thumbs, other fingers, pacifiers or other objects. It makes them feel secure and happy, and it helps them learn about their world. The prevalence of this habit is decreased as age increases, and mostly, it is stopped by 4 years of age. There is a relationship between the level of education in parents, the child nutrition and the sucking habit [17]. If the child chooses this habit in the first year of his or her life, the parents should move away his or her thumb smoothly and attract the child's attention to other things such as toys. After the second years of age, thumb sucking will decrease and will be appear just in child's bed or when he/she is tired. Some of children who do not stop this habit, will give it up when their permanent teeth erupt, but there is a tendency for continuing the sucking habit even until adult life. According to a study in 1973, millions of kids do not give up this habit before the eruption of teeth [18]. Nowadays, the level of stress is higher than the time of that study, and as stress is a powerful stimulus in sucking habit, it is probable to find more kids with long-term sucking habit if we do a research exactly like the one which was done in 1973.

Thumb sucking has 2 types:

1. Active: In this type, there is a heavy force by the muscles during the sucking and if this habit continues for a long period, the position of permanent teeth and the shape of mandible will be affected.

2. Passive: In this type, the child puts his/her finger in mouth, but because there is no force on teeth and mandible, so this habit is not associated with skeletal changes.

In the case of active thumb sucking habit, it is better for a child not to be blamed, teased, offended, humiliated and punished, because these methods will increase the anxiety and consequently increase the incidence of the habit. Long-term finger sucking habit has harmful effects on dentition and speech. In 1870s decade, Camble and Jander reported for the first time that long-term finger sucking has harmful effects on dentition [19].

The side effects of finger sucking are: Anterior open bite, increased overjet, lingual inclination lower incisor and labial inclination upper incisor, posterior cross bite, compensatory tongue thrust, deep palate, speech defect, and finger defects (Eczema of the finger due to alternate dryness and moisture that occurs and even angulations of the finger). The severity of changes in dentition due to finger sucking is related to the duration and times of doing the habit. Also, the position of finger in mouth, dental arches relation and child's health affect the severity of changes [20].

Dental changes due to finger sucking do not need any treatment if the habit stopped before the 5 years of age and as soon as giving up the habit, dental changes will be corrected spontaneously [21]. At the time of permanent anterior teeth eruption and if the child is motivated to stop the sucking habit, it is time to start the treatment as follows:

1. Direct interview with child if he/she is mature enough to understand

2. Encouragement: This can give the child more pride and self-confidence

3. Reward system

4. Reminder therapy

5. Orthodontic appliance: The final stage in treatment is the use of orthodontic appliance whether fixed or removable, which can play the role of reminder and can reduce the willing of finger sucking. For long-term habits or unwilling patient, the fixed intra oral appliance is the most effective inhibitor. In the case of using fixed or removable appliance, we should alarm the parents about potential problems in speaking or eating during the first 24 to 48 h, which are usual and self correcting. After active phase of treatment, the appliance should remain in place for more 3 to 6 month to minimize the relapse potential [22, 23].

5.2. Use of pacifier

The use of pacifier is common in most countries and it will not cause permanent changes in dentition if it is stopped at the age of 2 or 3 years. After that, the use of pacifier has harmful effects on dentition development, and if it is used more than 5 years old, these effects would be more severe [24]. The children who use pacifier are not willing to suck their fingers. pacifier has the following negative effects:

1. Anterior open bite

2. Shallow palate

3. Increased width of lower arch

4. Posterior cross bite.

5. Median otitis

It is suggested that pacifier should be replaced in children who have the habit of finger sucking, because the harmful effects of sucking pacifier are less than finger. In comparison between different pacifiers, despite the claims, it has been shown that there is no significant advantage for physiologic pacifiers over conventional ones [25].

5.3. Nail biting or onychophagia

Nail biting is a common and untreated medical problem among children. This habit starts after 3 to 4 years of age and is in its peak in 10 years of age. Its rate increases in adolescency, while it declines later. This problem is not gender dependent in children less than 10 years of age, but its incidence in boys is more than girls among adolescents [26]. This problem is a reaction in response to psychological disorders and some children will shift their habits from thumb sucking to nail biting. Complications caused by nail biting include malocclusion of the anterior teeth, teeth root resorption, bacterial infection and alveolar destruction. Moreover, about one forth of patients with temporo-mandibular joint pain and dysfunction have been shown to suffer from nail biting habit [27]. It is seen in clinic that boys with nail biting have a kind of psychological disorder especially attention deficient hyperactivity disorder (ADHD) more than girls. This habit in higher ages will be replaced with some habits such as lip chewing, gum chewing or smoking (Finn, 1998). Children with nail biting should be evaluated for emotional problems. In addition, putting nail polish or distasteful liquids on nails may be a therapeutic choice.

5.4. Tongue thrust

Tongue Thrust refers to a swallowing pattern in which the tongue is placed in the front of the mouth to begin the swallow (Fig. 5). Forward position of the tongue may also be seen at rest (mouth breathers). Normal swallowing patterns after infancy involve a coordinated smooth movement of the tongue toward the back of the mouth. This consistent forward movement of the tongue may cause speech errors and misaligned teeth. Forward positioning of the tongue during rest has the most influence on misaligning the teeth due to duration of the pressure. The speech disorder most commonly associated with tongue thrust is a frontal lisp, in which the tongue is place between the teeth for the sounds s and z, and sometimes for sh, ch, j, and soft g.

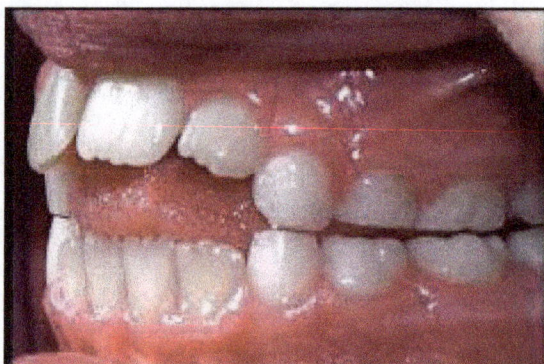

Figure 5. Tongue thrust

The line of treatment for these habits includes removal of the etiology, retraining exercises, and use of mechanical restraining appliances. Tongue bead appliances are commonly used as retraining exercise devices. In severe tongue thrusting cases and in cases with anterior open bite, a bead appliance alone may not be effective in restricting the habit. Tongue crib appliances (Fig. 6) are extremely effective in breaking the tongue thrust habit [28]. They create a mechanical barrier and prevent the tongue from thrusting between the incisors. In most of the cases with severe thumb/digit sucking habit, an anterior open bite develops. This will result in the development of a secondary tongue thrust habit. Hence, in cases with severe prolonged thumb or digit sucking, an appliance which can eliminate both of these habits. The Hybrid Habit Correcting Appliance (HHCA) can be used to effectively restrain and correct tongue thrusting as well as thumb sucking habit (Fig.7). HHCA incorporates a tongue bead, a palatal crib and a U-loop which is attached to the molar bands on either sides. The tongue bead consists of a spinnable acrylic bead of 3mm diameter. The appliance is designed to position the acrylic bead over the posterior one-third of the incisive papilla. The bead acts as a tongue retrainer. The patient is asked to constantly pull the bead towards the posterior region of the mouth. The palatal crib and the U-loop are made of 0.9mm stainless steel wire. Three to four spurs are bent on either sides of the bead, starting from the canine region on one side, running anteriorly as a smooth curve (in conventional crib appliances, the cribs run obliquely from one canine to the other side canine) and lying 1mm lingual to the cervical margin of the maxillary anterior teeth. In the region of the incisive papilla, the acrylic bead is incorporated in such a way that it lies over the posterior one-third of the incisive papilla. The tip of the crib should be almost in line with the incisor tip of the maxillary central incisor or 2 mm longer without interfering with the lower incisors when in occlusion. In cases with anterior open bite, the crib should be longer and can be up to 3/4th of the interincisal distance between the upper and lower central incisors. This is to avoid the tongue from thrusting over the tip of the crib. The palatal crib acts as a barrier against the thrusting tongue and works as a mechanical restrainer. The U-loop is incorporated in the second premolar region and it helps to reposition the appliance posteriorly during the retraction phase, when it is used along with fixed orthodontic appliances.

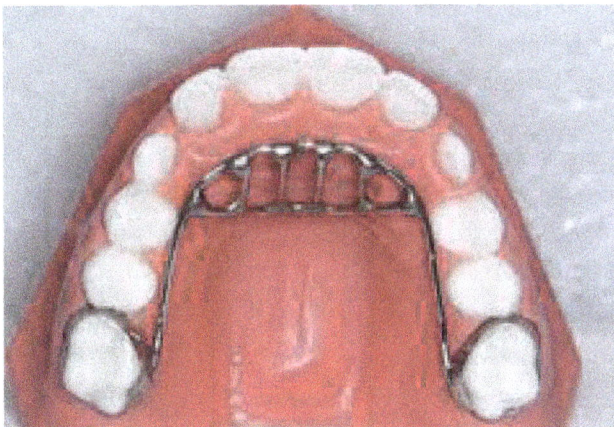

Figure 6. Tongue crib appliances

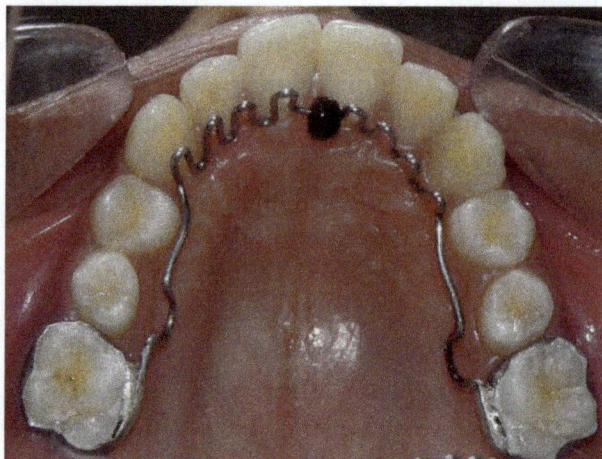

Figure 7. Hybrid Habit Correcting Appliance (HHCA).

5.5. Bruxism

The actions of masticatory system are divided into 2 groups. Functional actions such as mastication, speaking and swallowing, and parafunctional actions such as teeth impacting (clenching) and bruxism.

Functional activities are controllable and occurred daily. Parafunctional actions may be conscious or unconscious and are normally without sound. However, bruxism in nights is unconscious and mostly it is with sound production. Sleep bruxism occurs during stages first and second of non rapid eye movement (REM) sleep and REM sleep. These people do not have any complaint about bruxism, and it would not affect their quality of sleep. But in the old and people with sleep apnea, bruxism can reduce the quality of sleep [29]. Sleep bruxism has 2 types: Primary or idiopathic and secondary or iatrogenic. The first type is without any medical reason and the secondary type is whether with use of drug or without the use of drug. Risk factors are as follows: Genetics: 20 to 50% of patients with sleep bruxism have positive family history [30]; age: The prevalence of this habit decrease with age; cigarette smoking: The prevalence of sleep bruxism in smokers is 1.9 times more than non-smokers; use of alcohol and caffeine [31]; tension and stresses. Clinical findings of sleep bruxism include; report of grinding or impacting sounds of teeth; erosion of the teeth occlusal surfaces and breakdown of repairs; hypertrophy of masticatory muscles; hypersensitivity of teeth to cold air, and joint sounds. The treatment includes no special recommended regimen, but increasing awareness of the patient, intra oral appliances, behavioral treatment and drugs like diazepam and clonazepam have been reported to be effective [32,33].

6. Anterior cross bite correction

Anterior crossbite is defined as a malocclusion resulting from the lingual positioning of the maxillary anterior teeth in relationship to the mandibular anterior teeth. An anterior crossbite is present when one or more of the upper incisors are in linguo-occlusion (reverse over jet). This may involve just a single tooth or could include all four upper incisors. Anterior dental crossbite has a reported incidence of 4-5% and usually becomes evident during the early mixed-dentition phase [34]. Anterior crossbite correction in early mixed dentition is highly recommended as this kind of malocclusion does not diminish with age. Uncorrected anterior crossbite may lead to abnormal wear of the lower incisors, dental compensation of mandibular incisors leading to thinning of labial alveolar plate and/or gingival recession. However early treatment does not always eliminates orthodontic treatment need in permanent occlusion. The aim of early treatment of this type of malocclusion is to correct anterior crossbite, as otherwise often can lead to very serious Class III malocclusion which would be possible to treat only with combined orthodontic and orthognatic method.

A variety of factors has been reported to cause anterior dental crossbite, including a palatal eruption path of the maxillary anterior incisors; trauma to the primary incisor resulting in lingual displacement of the permanent tooth germ; supernumerary anterior teeth; an over-retained necrotic or pulpless deciduous tooth or root; odontomas; crowding in the incisor region; inadequate arch length; and a habit of biting the upper lip. Various treatment methods have been proposed to correct anterior dental crossbite, such as tongue blades, reversed stainless steel crowns, fixed acrylic planes, bonded resin-composite slopes, and removable acrylic appliances with finger springs.

Bayraka and Tunca, 2008, described the use of bonded resin-composite slopes for the management of anterior crossbite in children in early mixed dentition. Dental crossbite was corrected by applying a 3-4 mm bonded resin-composite slope to the incisal edge of the mandibular incisor with an angle 45° to the longitudinal axis of the tooth (Fig. 8). Correction was achieved within 1-2 weeks with no damage to either the tooth or the marginal periodontal tissue. The procedure was a simple and effective method for treating anterior dental crossbite [35].

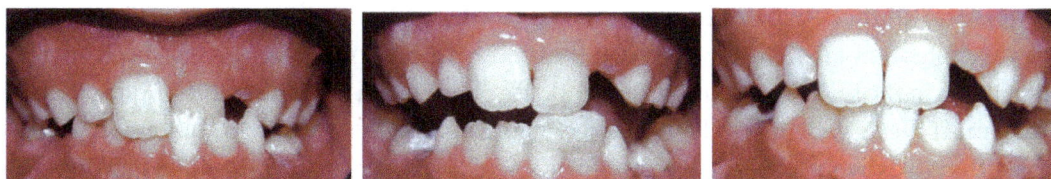

Figure 8. Anterior crossbite correction with bonded resin-composite slope

Some authors believe that removable appliances are not preferred in anterior crossbite correction as they tend to get displaced as the turning frequency decreases following activation. Moreover, poor patient compliance with removable appliance can cause relapse of the case and poor success rate. Therefore, a fixed appliance was proposed as a more sound therapy. Yaseen and Acharya, 2012, described the use of hexa helix, a modified version of quad helix for the management of anterior crossbite and bilateral posterior crossbite in early mixed dentition (Fig. 9). Correction was achieved within 15 weeks with no damage to the tooth or the marginal periodontal tissue. The procedure is a simple and effective method for treating anterior and bilateral posterior crossbite simultaneously. it provides advantages such as minimal discomfort, reduces need for patient cooperation, and better control of tooth movements [36].

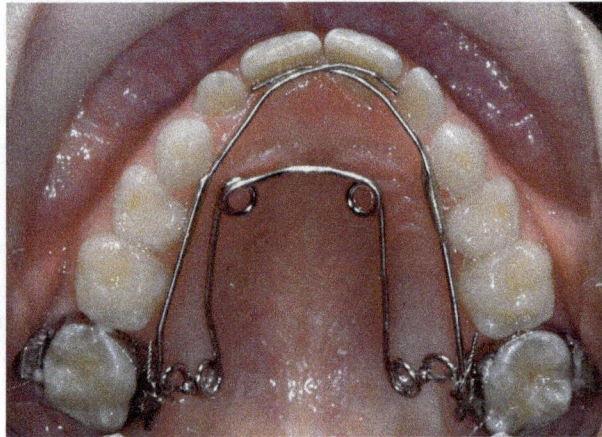

Figure 9. Hexa helix appliance.

In a recent study, Wiedel and Bondemark, 2014, evaluated and compared the stability of correction of anterior crossbite in the mixed dentition by fixed or removable appliance therapy. The study comprised 64 consecutive patients who met the following inclusion criteria: early to late mixed dentition, anterior crossbite affecting one or more incisors, no inherent skeletal Class III discrepancy, moderate space deficiency, a nonextraction treatment plan, and no previous orthodontic treatment. The study was designed as a randomized controlled trial with two parallel arms. The patients were randomized for treatment with a removable appliance with protruding springs or with a fixed appliance with multi-brackets. The outcome measures were success rates for crossbite correction, overjet, overbite, and arch length. Measurements were made on study casts before treatment (T0), at the end of the retention period (T1), and 2 years after retention (T2). Results showed that at T1 the anterior crossbite had been corrected in all patients in the fixed appliance group and all except one in the removable appliance group. At T2, almost all treatment results remained stable and equal in both groups. From T0 to T1, minor differences were observed between the fixed and removable appliance groups with respect to changes in overjet, overbite, and arch length measurements. These changes had no clinical implications and remained unaltered at T2. It was concluded that in the mixed dentition, anterior crossbite affecting one or more incisors can be successfully corrected by either fixed or removable appliances with similar long-term stability [37].

7. Anterior diastema and abnormal labial fraenum

Angle described the midline diastema as a common form of incomplete occlusion character-ized by a space between the maxillary and, less frequently, mandibular central incisors. In his classical article, Andrews stated that interdental diastemas should not exist and all contacts should be tight so that the patient has 'straight and attractive teeth as well as a correct overall dental occlusion'.

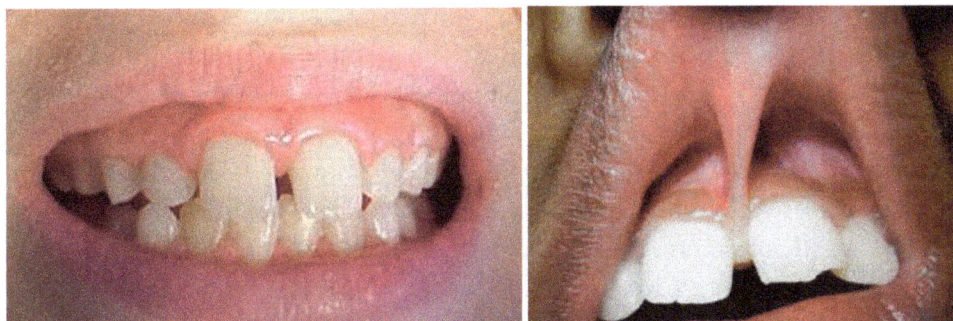

Figure 10. Midline diastema

Sanin et al., developed a method that could predict whether the space would close spontaneously in the developing dentition. This method is based on millimeter measurements in the early mixed dentition and is claimed to have an accuracy of 88%. As the size of the diastema increases the possibility of space closure without treatment reduces. Sanin's prediction is as follows:

* For a 1 mm space in the early mixed dentition the possibility of spontaneous space closure is 99%.

* For a 1.5 mm space the possibility is 85%.

* For a 1.85 mm diastema it is 50%.

* For a 2.7 mm space the possibility of closure without treatment is only 1%.

The measurement should be made after the eruption of the lateral incisors. Hence it is advisable to intervene early if the midline diastema is more than 1.85 mm after the eruption of the permanent lateral incisors [38].

To treat the midline diastema effectively, an accurate diagnosis of the etiology and an intervention relevant to the specific etiology is necessary. Timing of the treatment is important to achieve satisfactory results. Most of the researchers do not recommend tooth movement until the eruption of the permanent canines, but in certain cases, where very large diastemas exist, treatment can be initiated early [39].

Nainar and Gnanasundaram noted in their study of midline diastemas on 9774 Southern Indian individuals, that there was a relatively increased frequency of familial occurrence and hence proposed the presence of a genetic factor in the expression of midline diastema. Treatment methods include orthodontic correction with a fixed or removable appliance and prosthetic correction with composites and crowns. If the diastema is large, it is advisable to close the space using orthodontic appliances. In most cases, simple removable appliances incorporating finger springs or a split labial bow can give good results [40].

A hypertrophic labial frenum may be considered as a major etiological factor for midline diastema. In a thick and fleshy labial frenum, the fibro-elastic band crosses the alveolus and inserts into the incisive papilli, preventing the approximation of the maxillary central incisors. The blanching test is a simple diagnostic test to predict whether a normal tight contact between the central incisors. Most of the researchers, like Angle, Sicher, and Edwards, [41-43] are of the opinion that superior labial frenum causes midline diastema. Some researchers, like Popovich et al, believe that there is an inverse relationship between high frenal attachment and midline diastema. According to them, labial frenum persists owing to the existing diastema and, as the dentition applies little or no pressure on the tissues, here is little or no atrophy of the frenum [44]. However, most of the researchers agree that removal of the high bulbous labial frenum is important for the stability after the closure of the midline diastema.

Excessive anterior overbite is another major contributing factor for midline diastema. As a result of trauma to the maxillary anterior teeth from the mandibular incisors, the maxillary incisors procline. This results in an increase of the upper arch circumference, leading to a diastema. Practitioners should not fail to identify deep bite as an aetiology for the diastema. Any attempt to close the midline spacing without correcting the deep bite and anterior traumatic bite will lead to a speedy relapse of the condition.

Oral habits such as tongue thrusting and finger sucking can be other etiological factors for the appearance of the midline diastema. According to Proffit and Fields, tongue position at rest may have a greater impact on tooth position than tongue pressure, as the tongue only briefly contacts the lingual surface of the anterior teeth during thrusting [45]. The tongue pushes the anterior teeth to a forward position, increasing the circumference which results in spacing. An abnormal habit of the tongue can be detected by the tip of the tongue popping out through the anterior spacing when the patient is asked to swallow. In cases of anterior open bite, the tongue may be seen thrusting between incisal edges of the maxillary and mandibular incisors. Patients with tongue thrust often produce a snap sound on swallowing and also have hyperactivity of the orbicularis oris muscle.Deleterious habits have to be corrected by using habit-breaking appliances and by psychological approaches. The use of fixed tongue cribs are found to be effective in breaking the tongue-thrusting habit.

Peg-shaped laterals Supernumerary teeth/mesiodens, missing teeth, pathologic migration of teeth Tooth size, arch size discrepancy, angulation of teeth, odontomas occurring in the maxillary midline, developmental cysts in the orofacial midline, and flaccid lips are other proposed etiological factors leading to midline diastema. Relapse is a major concern in the correction of midline diastema. However, exact diagnosis and removal of the etiology is the key to obtaining a stable result. Long-term use of retainers or even permanent bonded lingual retainers are advocated, especially in cases with large diastema. Large pre-treatment diastema presence of at least one family member with a similar condition increases the risk of relapse [46,47].

8. Serial extraction

The term serial extraction describes an orthodontic treatment procedure that involves the orderly removal of selected deciduous and permanent teeth in a predetermined sequence (Dewel, 1969). Serial extraction can be defined as the correctly timed, planned removal of certain deciduous and permanent teeth in mixed dentition cases with dento-alveolar dispro-portion in order to: Alleviate crowding of incisor teeth and to allow unerupted teeth to guide themselves into improved positions (canines in particular), and to lessen (or eliminate) the period of active appliance therapy. Thus, it is one of the positive interceptive orthodontic procedure generally applied in most discrepancy cases where supporting bone is less than the total tooth material [48].

Serial extraction has been of interest to dentist for many years. Throughout the history of dentistry it has been recognized that the removal of one or more irregular teeth would improve the appearance of the reminder. Nance presented clinics on his technique of progressive extraction in 1940 and has been called as the father of serial extraction philosophy in the United States. Kjellgren in 1940 termed this extraction procedure as planned or progressive extraction procedure of teeth. Hotz, 1970, named the same procedure on "Guidance of eruption". According to him the term guidance of eruption is comprehensive and encompasses all measures available for influencing tooth eruption [49]. Widespread adoption of serial extrac-tion as a corrective treatment procedure continues to be a source of concern to all pedodontists who are aware of its limitations as well as of its possibilities. The principle reason is that its application involves growth prediction. Every serial extraction diagnosis is based on the promise that future growth will be inadequate to accommodate all of the teeth in a normal alignment.

If primary teeth are extracted prematurely, this will influence the eruption rate and position of the permanent successors. In general, the eruption will be delayed if the primary tooth overlying the permanent tooth is extracted 1 ½ years or more from the time the primary tooth would normally exfoliate. Conversely, the eruption rate can be accelerated if the primary tooth overlying the permanent tooth is extracted less than a year before the primary tooth would normally exfoliate. Biologic variation in eruption rates will affect these time tables, as will periapical inflammation of the primary tooth. Another useful principle is that crowded teeth adjacent to an extraction site tend to align themselves [50].

Normal dental, skeletal and profile development – influences the rationale for serial extraction. The work of Moorrees et al on arch dimensions and serial extractions indicates that there is minimal increase in mandibular intercanine width between 8 and 18 years, occurring usually around the time the permanent mandibular canines erupt. The maxillary intercanine width increases slightly more and over a longer time. The dental arch perimeter from the distal of the mandibular primary second molar to its antimere is less in the permanent dentition than in the primary. Also the principles of leeway space, interrelationship of overjet, overbite, axial inclinations, and mesial shift, and arch-length analysis must be considered in determining whether to institute a serial extraction procedure. The skeletal and profile factors that influence serial extractions are the another-posterior, vertical, and transverse relationships as well as the developmental pattern. Specifically the relation of the maxilla to the mandible and of the both to the cranial base must be determined to identify protrusions, retrusions, hyperdivergences, hypodivergences, crossbites, and asymmetries. Also rotational, vertical, and transverse growth patterns need to be integrated into the decision-making process [51].

The idea of serial extraction started when Pedodontist sees a child 5 or 6 years of age with all the deciduous teeth present in a slightly crowded state or with no spaces between them, he can predict, with a fair degree of certainly, that there will not be enough space in the jaws to accommodate all the permanent teeth in their proper alignment. As Nance (1940), Dewel (1954), and others have pointed out, after the eruption of the first permanent molars at 6 years of age, there is probably no increase in the distance from the mesial aspect of the first molar on one side around the arch to the mesial aspect of the first molar on the opposite side. If there is any change, it may be an actual reduction of the molar-to-molar arch length, as the "leeway" space is lost through the mesial migration of the first permanent molars during the tooth-exchange process and correction of the flush terminal plane relationship. At that time, a list of possible clinical clues for serial extraction were proposed: Premature loss of deciduous teeth, arch-length deficiency and tooth size discrepancies, lingual eruption of lateral incisors, unilateral deciduous canine loss and shift to the same side, mesial eruption of canines overlateral incisors, mesial drift of buccal segments, abnormal eruption direction and eruption sequence, flaring of incisors, ectopic eruption of mandibular first deciduous molar, abnormal resorption of II deciduous molar, ankylosis, labial stripping, and gingival recession, usually of lower incisor. However, a number of contraindications for serial extractions were addressed: Congenital absence of teeth providing space, mild to moderate crowding, deep or open bites, severe Class II, III of dental/skeletal origin, cleft lip and palate, spaced dentition, anodontia / oligodontia, Midline diastemia, dilacerations extensive caries, disportion between arc length and tooth material.

9. Considerations in serial extraction

1. Extracting primary canines will produce maximum amounts of self improvement in crowding with greatest inter-ception of lingual cross bite.

2. Extracting primary first molars produces earliest eruption of first premolars but reduces speed and amount of improvement in permanent central and lateral incisors crowding and position due to retention of C that it has limited application.

3. Extracting primary canines and first molars is a compromise between rapid improvement in and desired early eruption of permanent central and lateral incisors due to simultaneous eruption of first premolars with this extraction sequence.

There is no single technique for Serial Extraction. It is a long-range guidance program and it may be necessary to reevaluate and change tentative decisions several times. Usually the child is 7-8 years of age when he/she brought to the pedodontist. At this time the maxillary and mandibular central incisors are usually erupted, but there is inadequate space in anterior segments to allow normal eruption and positioning of lateral incisors. In some cases, mandibular lateral incisors have already erupted but they are usually lingually positioned and rotated. The same is with the maxillary lateral incisors.

9.1. Dewel's method

There are 3 stages in Serial Extraction Therapy:

First: Removal of deciduous canines : to permit eruption and optimal alignment of lateral incisors. There is some amount of improvement in position of central incisors also.

Second: Removal of first deciduous molars: to accelerate eruption of first premolars ahead of canine if possible.

Third: Removal of erupting first premolars: Before the first premolars are extracted, all the diagnostic criteria must again be evaluated. The status of developing third molars must be evaluated, because if the third molars are congenitally missing then extraction of 1st premolars would be unnecessary because there would be enough space. So in short, Dewel's method is:

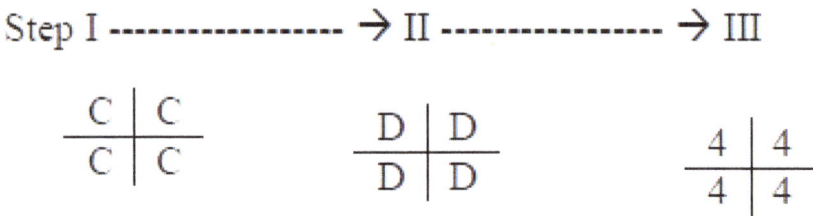

$$\text{Step I} \dashrightarrow \text{II} \dashrightarrow \text{III}$$

$$\frac{C \mid C}{C \mid C} \qquad \frac{D \mid D}{D \mid D} \qquad \frac{4 \mid 4}{4 \mid 4}$$

9.2. Tweed's method

According to Tweed, if diagnosis shows the discrepancy exists between teeth and basal bone structures and if patient is between 7 ½ to 8 ½ years, Serial Extraction program is should be carried out. Sequence is:

First: At approximately 8 years all deciduous molars are extracted. It is preferable to maintain in deciduous canines to retard eruption of permanent canines.

Second: extract of first premolar and deciduous canines should he done 4-6 months prior to eruption of permanent canines when they erupt they migrate posteriorly into good position. Any irregularities in mandibular incisors if not too severe, get corrected themselves and they are also tipped lingually due to normal muscular forces.

9.3. Moyers method

Proposed when crowding seen in central incisor region. Fairly eruption of lateral incisors.

Stage I (Extraction of all deciduous lateral incisors). It helps in alignment of central incisors.

Stage II (Extraction of all deciduous canines after 7-8 months). It helps in alignment of lateral incisors and provides space for lateral incisors.

Stage III (Extraction of all deciduous first molars). It stimulates eruption of all first premolars.

Stage IV (Extraction of all first premolars after 7-8 months). It provides space for canines and stimulates eruption of canines.

Step I ----------- → II ------------ → III ------------ → IV

$$\frac{B \mid B}{B \mid B} \qquad \frac{C \mid C}{C \mid C} \qquad \frac{D \mid D}{D \mid D} \qquad \frac{4 \mid 4}{4 \mid 4}$$

The technique of serial extraction was biologically sound proven, and was not considered a compromise. with continuous observation and study, the sight has changed. conventional orthodontic therapy is required to complete the alignment of teeth, to parallel the roots on either side, of the extraction space, to eliminate overbite, and to effect residual space closure. With advances in fixed orthodontics, less damage and more stable results are obtained. Moreover, it must be remembered that, once teeth have been extracted, they cannot be replaced if an error in judgment must be made, it is more expedient to error in a conservative manner without extraction as teeth can always be extracted at a later date. To summarize the limitations a and side effects of serial extraction:

First: Tendency of bite to close following loss of posterior teeth. A normal overbite depends on adequate vertical growth and Serial Extraction involves removal of strategically located deciduous and permanent teeth. Vertical and horizontal growth depends great part on normal proximal and occlusal function in maintaining arch length and normal overjet and overbite.

Second: Failure of premolars that fail to reach their normal occlusal level. In normally developing dentition, the premolars are ready to emerge soon after the loss of the deciduous molars and then proceed occlusally with no delay. But in Serial Extraction cases the premolars have to travel a long way before penetrating the gingival tissues. Prolonged absence of teeth in the posterior segment of arches permits the tongue to flow into remaining spaces and this may remain as a tongue thrusting habit. This in turn prevents premolars from attaining full eruption.

Third: Effect of serial extraction on facial esthetics. Most of us over emphasize on straight profile which has led to extraction of teeth in mixed dentition because the lips appear to be prominent. Its normal for lip line to have greater convexity during early transitional stages than it will have in mature dentition. Lip fullness is not a reliable criterion for extraction in early mixed dentition. The straight profile must be viewed with greater concern because early removal of premolars is likely to cause a concave profile.

Fourth: Nasal development is another unpredictable hazard. The nose is one structure that continues to grow long after other facial parts have reached maturity. Unrestrained extraction will accentuate its prominence by reducing skeletal development in dental area. Moreover growth of chin is unpredictable. If growth in nose and chin exceeds normal range a concave profile is obtained.

In conclusion, one team of clinicians and practioners demonstrate that undertaking a serial extraction protocol can afforded an improvement of the patient's self-esteem, resulting in a positive social impact due to esthetic enhancement. Furthermore, the low cost of this protocol permits the use of this therapy in underprivileged communities provided the diagnosis is certain and the post extraction movement of teeth is controlled by mechanical means. The other team suggest that serial extraction is counter-productive. The early extraction of primary cuspids will invariably result in crowding of the permanent cuspids region. In reality, they adopt the idea that the problem is maintained and the crowding shifts to involve the permanent cuspids. They remind us with the most basic canon of the health profession which is "first do no harm" [52].

10. Interceptive functional therapy

There is little doubt that functional appliances produce tooth movement and in many cases can correct occlusal discrepancies. The controversy over their use relates mainly to their mode of action, and in particular to two aspects. The first is the question of modification of growth of the basal parts of the jaws. Many authorities believe that basal jaw growth can be altered by functional means. The temporo-mandibular joint area has been thought to be a reactive growth site, i.e. any prolonged change in the position of the mandible during the growth period, such as is induced by wearing the appliance, results in bone apposition on the mandibular and temporal surfaces of the enlarged joint cavity. Baume, (1969) quotes histological evidence to support this concept, and ample clinical evidence has been produced in attempts to show that the use of functional appliances can alter the skeletal relationship of the jaws [53]. On the other hand, this clinical evidence does not always take into account the effects of normal growth. As functional appliances are normally used during the mixed dentition stage a considerable amount of normal growth must occur which could alter jaw size and relationships. Several investigators have failed to find evidence of altered growth with functional appliances, but instead have found the main effects to be tipping of the incisors and an opening rotation of the mandible [54,55].

The first practitioner to use functional jaw orthopedics to treat a malocclusion was Pierre Robin (1902).

His appliance influenced muscular activity by changing the spatial relationship of the jaws. Robin's monoloc was actually a modification of Kingsley's maxillary plate. It extended all along the lingual surfaces of the mandibular teeth, but it had sharp lingual imprints of the crown surfaces of both maxillary and mandibular teeth. It incorporated an expansion screw in the palate to expand the dental arches. In 1909, Viggo Andresen, a Danish dentist, used lingual horseshoe flange that guides the mandible forward to eliminate Class II malocclusion cases. The original Andresen activator was a tooth-borne, loosely fitting passive appliance consisting of a block of plastic covering the palate and the teeth of both arches, designed to advance the mandible several millimeters for Class II correction and open the bite 3 to 4 mm. The original design had facets incorporated into the body of the appliance to direct erupting posterior teeth mesially or distally, so, despite the simple design, dental relationships in all 3 planes of space could be changed.

The Herbst appliance (Dentaurum, Newtown, Pa) is suitable for slightly older children whose cooperation might not be dependable, because it is a fixed appliance worn 24 hours a day. The Herbst was introduced in 1905 by Emil Herbst, but his findings were not published until 1935. Little more was published on the appliance until the late 1970s, when Hans Pancherz, recognizing its possibilities for mandibular growth stimulation, revived interest. The typical Herbst consists of a telescoping mechanism connected to the maxillary first molars at one end and a cantilevered arm attached to the mandibular first molars at the other end; it forces the mandible forward (Fig. 11).

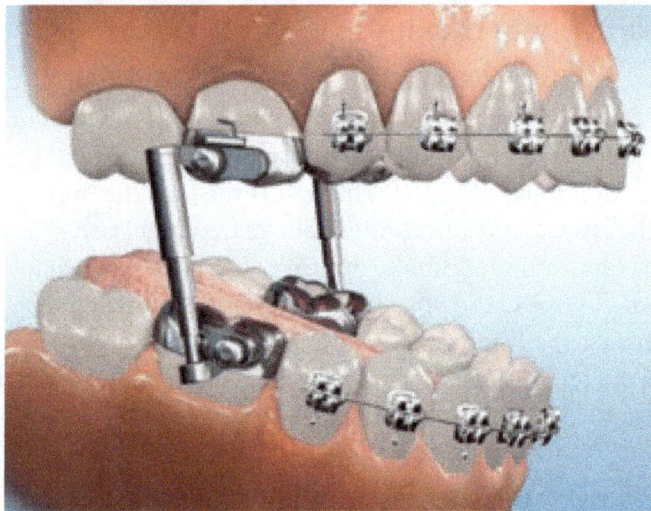

Figure 11. Herbst Appliance

In 1950, Wilhelm Balters (1893-1973), in an effort to treat Class II malocclusions characterized by deficient mandibles, began to modify Andresen's activator. He gave it the name bionator. It is indicated for patients with favorable facial growth patterns and is designed to produce forward positioning of the mandible. As with the function regulator, the bionator is available in 3 designs. Consisting of 2 halves connected by a Coffin spring, it is less restrictive of speech than Andresen's appliance. However, the treatment also highly depends on patient compliance, especially with regard to exercising

The Clark twin-block (Clark 1988) consists of separate upper and lower removable appliances, each with a 45° posterior bite plane designed to induce a mandibular posture of the desired amount and direction (Fig. 12) One or both sections may incorporate a mid-line screw to effect arch expansion(Fig. 13), and there is provision for the addition of extraoral traction.

Many clinical studies have been done on skeletal and dentoalveolar changes associated with functional appliances therapy in Class II malocclusions, but the scientific data are still controversial. Concerning skeletal effects induced by the functional appliances some authors

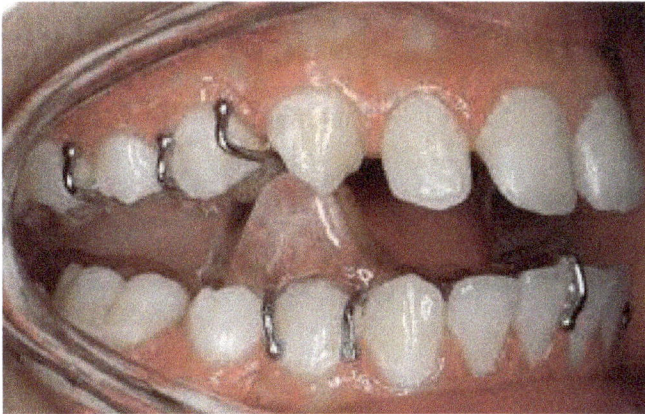

Figure 12. Twin-block appliance

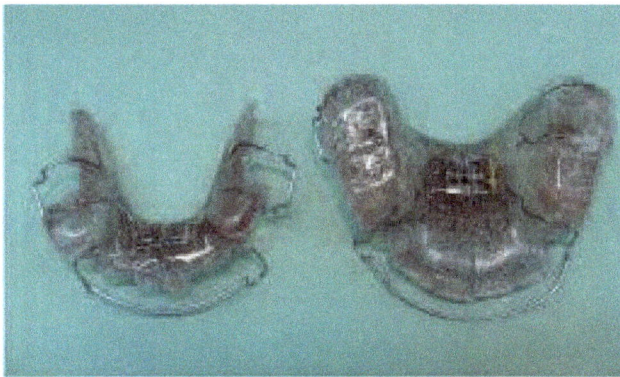

Figure 13. Expansion screw within Twin block appliance

demonstrate significant influences on mandibular growth [56], the others claim that it may be induced only small skeletal changes by this type of treatment [57]. The latter group of researchers found that the main changes occurred with functional appliance therapy were dentoalveolar distalization of the buccal and retroclination of the frontal upper teeth, along with mesial movement of the lower buccal segments and proclination of the lower labial segments[58]. Such diversity of results on skeletal changes might be related first of all to difficulties in applying treatment at the maximum growth spurt time. Another reason for the inconsistence in assessment of treatment results might be the use of not reliable reference lines and/or structures for cephalometric analysis before and after treatment. This makes difficult to assess real contribution of skeletal and dental components to occlusal changes [59]. A new paradigm for successful treatment presents a philosophical challenge to combine the benefits of orthodontic and orthopedic techniques to extend our horizons in the treatment of malocclusion that requires dental and skeletal correction.

The prefabricated myofunctional appliances are a series of prefabricated appliances produced by myoresearch company, Queensland, Australia. These appliances were also called "Trainers™" which include T4K™ and T4F™ appliances (Fig.14,15). The idea of prefabricated functional appliances was recently introduced to the orthodontic field and it becomes more practical with the new customizable functional appliance T4F™. The T4F™ appliance is a prefabricated re-mouldable appliance when immersed in very hot water so it can be customized to accommodate the patient's dentition in the mouth and increase the retention. This new functional appliance has the advantage of the immediate issuing and the direct fitting of the appliance in the patient's mouth and it is also a better choice in terms of the cost for the private practitioners. The prefabricated appliances were claimed to be effective for class II Div.1 management but there was no evidence except for T4K™ type which is designed for young children.

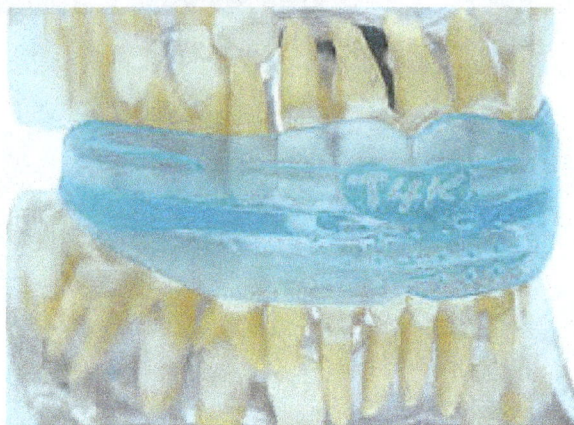

Figure 14. T4K™ The Pre-Orthodontic Trainer

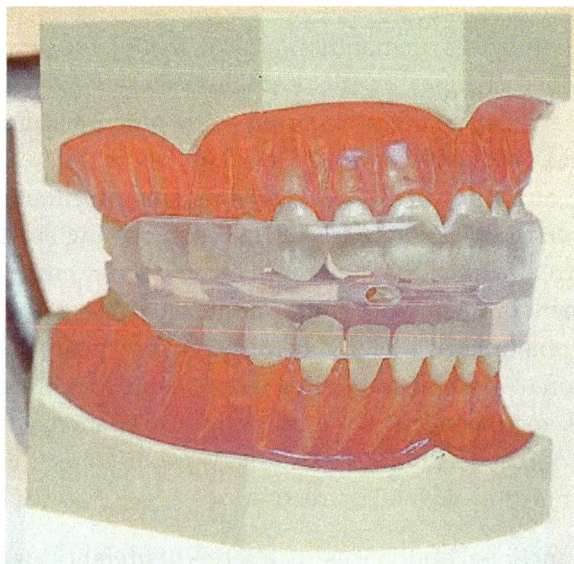

Figure 15. T4F™ The Pre-Orthodontic Trainer

Uysal et al., 2012, evaluated the effects of Pre-Orthodontic Trainer (T4F™) appliance on the anterior temporal, mental, orbicularis oris, and masseter muscles through electromyography (EMG) evaluations in subjects with Class II division 1 malocclusion and incompetent lips. Twenty patients (mean age: 9.8 ± 2.2 years) with a Class II division 1 malocclusion were treated with T4F™ (Myofunctional Research Co., Queensland, Australia). A group of 15 subjects (mean age: 9.2 ± 0.9 years) with untreated Class II division 1 malocclusions was used as a control. EMG recordings of treatment group were taken at the beginning and at the end of the T4F™ therapy (mean treatment period: 7.43 ± 1.06 months). Follow-up records of the control group were taken after 8 months of the first records. Recordings were taken during different oral functions: clenching, sucking, and swallowing. Statistical analyses were undertaken with Wilcoxon and Mann-Whitney U-tests. During the T4F™ treatment, activity of anterior temporal, mental, and masseter muscles was decreased and orbicularis oris activity was increased during clenching and these differences were found statistically significant when compared to control. Orbicularis oris activity during sucking was increased in the treatment group ($P < 0.05$). In the control group, significant changes were determined for anterior temporal ($P < 0.05$) and masseter ($P < 0.01$) muscle at clenching and orbicularis oris muscle at swallowing during observation period ($P < 0.05$). Findings indicated that treatment with T4F™ appliance showed a positive influence on the masticatory and perioral musculature [60].

Usumez et al., 2004, evaluated the dentoskeletal treatment effects induced by a preorthodontic trainer appliance (T4K™) treatment on Class II, division 1 cases. Twenty patients (10 girls and 10 boys, mean age 9.6+/-1.3 years) with a Class II, division 1 malocclusion were treated with T4K™ (Myofunctional Research Co., Queensland, Australia). The patients were instructed to use the trainer every day for one hour and overnight while they slept. A control group of 20 patients (mean age 10.2+/-0.8 years) with untreated Class II, division 1 malocclusions was used to eliminate possible growth effects. Lateral cephalograms were taken at the start and end of treatment. Final cephalograms were taken 13.1+/-1.8 months after trainer application, compared with a mean of 11.2+/-2.4 months later for the control group. The mean and standard deviations for cephalometric measurements were analyzed by paired-samples t-test and independent-samples t-tests. At the end of the study period, the trainer group subjects showed significant changes including anterior rotation and sagittal growth of the mandible, increased SNB and facial height, reduced ANB, increased lower incisor proclination, retroclination of upper incisors, and overjet reduction. However, only total facial height increase, lower incisor proclination, and overjet reduction were significantly higher when compared with the changes observed in the control group. This study was the first that demonstrated that the preorthodontic trainer application induces basically dentoalveolar changes that result in significant reduction of overjet and can be used with appropriate patient selection [61].

In a very recent study, Dr. Hanoun and his colleagues evaluated the effectiveness of the pre-fabricated myofunctional appliance T4F™ (compared to Twin Block appliance) in the treatment of Class II Div.1 malocclusion. The study was a prospective randomized clinical trial. All subjects were growing patients aged 11 -14 years old with Class II Div.1 malocclusion based on Class II skeletal relationship with overjet of 7 mm or more. Those subjects who had anterior open bite or previous orthodontic therapy or craniofacial anomalies or history of facial trauma were all excluded from the trial. The overjet was reduced more favourably in the Twin Block group than in the T4F™ group with a mean difference between the two groups of 2.14 mm (p <0.01). Moreover, there was a significant difference between both groups in terms of horizontal skeletal linear dimensions of the mandible with more favourable increase in the Twin Block group (p < 0.05).

11. Conclusion

Interceptive orthodontics is employed to recognize and eliminate potential irregularities and malposition in the developing dentofacial complex. These procedures are directed to lessen or to eliminate the severity of developing malocclusion. The early assessment of the child, followed by regular review, and treatment at the appropriate time if necessary, will do much to reduce malocclusion to the basic non-preventable level. The key to prevention of this kind is awareness. This part examines the key areas relating to interceptive orthodontics with the available evidence to support the clinical management of common problems presenting in the mixed dentition.

Acknowledgements

I offer my sincerest gratitude to my wife, Mrs. Huda Zurigat who has supported me throughout my project with a lot of patience and enthusiasm. Her assistance in typing and organizing words and figures in this article was indispensible.

Author details

Maen H. Zreaqat*

Address all correspondence to: maenzreqat@yahoo.com

Al-Ogaly Medical Group, Saudi Arabia

References

[1]   Weinberger BW. Historical résumé of the evolution and growth of orthodontia. J Am Dent Assoc 1934;21:201-221.

[2]   Asbell MB. A brief history of orthodontics. Am J Orthod Dentofacial Orthop 1990;98:176-83.

[3] Casto FM. A historical sketch of orthodontia. Dent Cosmos 1934;76:111-35.

[4] Brodie AG. Orthodontic history and what it teaches. Angle Orthod 1934;4:85-97.

[5] Irurita J, Alemán I, López-Lázaro S, Viciano J, Botella MC. Chronology of the development of the deciduous dentition in Mediterranean population. Forensic Sci Int. 2014;240:95-103.

[6] Borrie F, Bonetti D, Bearn D. What influences the implementation of interceptive orthodontics in primary care? Br Dent J. 2014;216(12):687-91.

[7] Kerosuo H1, Väkiparta M, Nyström M, Heikinheimo K. The seven-year outcome of an early orthodontic treatment strategy. J Dent Res. 2008;87(6):584-8.

[8] Norman W. Orthodontics in 3 millennia. Chapter 12: Two controversies: Early treatment and occlusion Am J Orthod Dentofacial Orthop. 2006;130(6):799-804.

[9] Baroni C; Franchini A; Rimondini L: Survival of different types of space maintainers. Pediatr Dent. 1994;16:360-61.

[10] Kirzioglu Z, Ozay MS Z, Ozay MS. Success of reinforced fibre material space maintainers. J Dent Child. 2004;71;2:158-62.

[11] Kargul B, Caglar E, Kabalay U. Glass fibre reinforced composite resin as fixed space maintainer in children 12 month clinical follow up. J Dent Child. 2005; 72(3):109-12

[12] Kargul B, Çaglar E, Kabalay U. Glass fiber-reinforced composite resin space maintainer: case reports. J Dent Child. 2003;71:258-61.

[13] Goldberg AJ, Frelich MA. Tooth splinting and stabilisation Dent Clin North Am. 1999; 43 (1) :127-33.

[14] Setia V, Pandit IK, Srivastava N, Gugnani N, Sekhon HK. Space maintainers in dentistry: past to present. J Clin Diagn Res. 2013;7(10):2402-5.

[15] Kharbanda O. P, Sidhu S. S, Sundaram K, Shukla D. K, "Oral habits in school going children of Delhi: a prevalence study," Journal of the Indian Society of Pedodontics and Preventive Dentistry. 2003; 21 (3): 120–124.

[16] Larson EF. The prevalence and etiology of prolonged dumy and finger sucking habit. Am. J. Orthod., 1985; 87(5):172-174.

[17] Farsi NM, Salama FS.. Sucking habits in Saudi children: prevalence, contributing factors and effects on the primary dentition. Pediatr. Dent. 1997; 19(1):28-33.

[18] N. L. Villa, "Changes in the dentition secondary to palatal crib therapy in digit-suckers: a preliminary study," Pediatric Dentistry, vol. 19, no. 5, pp. 323–326, 1997.

[19] B. S. Haskell and J. R. Mink, "An aid to stop thumb sucking: the "Bluegrass" appliance," Pediatric Dentistry. 1991; 13 (2): 83– 85.

[20] Van Norman RA (1997). Digit-sucking: A review of the literature, clinical observations and treatment recommendations. Int. J. Orofacial Myol., 23: 14-34

[21] Warren JJ, Bishara SE (2002). Duration of nutritive and nonnutritive sucking behavior and their effects on the dental arches in the primary dentition. Am. J. Orthod., 121: 347-356.

[22] Moimaz SA, Garbin AJ, Lima AM, Lolli LF, Saliba O, Garbin CA. Longitudinal study of habits leading to malocclusion development in childhood. BMC Oral Health. 2014; (4):14-96.

[23] Maia-Nader M, Silva de Araujo Figueiredo C, Pinheiro de Figueiredo F, Moura da Silva AA, Thomaz EB, Saraiva MC, Barbieri MA, Bettiol H. Factors associated with prolonged non-nutritive sucking habits in two cohorts of Brazilian children. BMC Public Health. 2014;14:14-17.

[24] Fleming PJ, Blaive PS Pacifier use an sudden infant death syndrome. Arch. Dis. Children. 1999; 81(2): 112-116.

[25] Lopes TS, Moura Lde F, Lima MC. Breastfeeding and sucking habits in children enrolled in a mother-child health program. BMC Res Notes. 2014;14(7): 23-38.

[26] Tanaka OM, Vitral RW, Tanaka GY, Guerrero AP, Camargo ES. (. Nailbiting, or onychophagia: A special habit. Am. J. Orthod. Dentofacial Orthop. 2008;134(2): 305-308.

[27] Saheeb D. Prevalence of oral and parafunctional habits in Nigerian patients suffering temporomandibular joint pain and dysfunftion. J. Med. Biomed. Res., (2005; 4(1): 59-64

[28] Feu D1, Menezes LM, Quintão AP, Quintão CC. A customized method for palatal crib fabrication. J Clin Orthod. 2013 Jul;47(7):406-12.

[29] Kato T, Thein NMR, Montplaisir JY, Lavigne GJ. Bruxism and orofacial movements during sleep. Dent. Clin. North Am. 2001;45(4):651-676.

[30] Hublin C, Kaprio J, Partinen M, Koskenvuo M. Sleep bruxism based on self – report in a nationwide twin cohort. Sleep Res. 1998;7(1): 61-68

[31] Dahan JS, Lelong BA, Celant S, Leysen V. Oral perception in tounge thrust and other oral habits. Am. J. Orthod. Dentofacial Orthop., 2000;118:385-91.

[32] Pierce CJ, Gale EN. A comparison of different treatments for nocturnal bruxism. J. Dent. Res., 1988;67: 597-601.

[33] Ferreira NM, Dos Santos JF, Dos Santos MB, Marchini L. Sleep bruxism associated with obstructive sleep apnea syndrome in children. Cranio. 2014 Sep [Epub ahead of print].

[34] Major PW, Glover K. Treatment of anterior cross-bites in the early mixed dentition. Journal of the Canadian Dental Association. 1992;58(7):574–578.

[35] Bayrak S1, Tunc ES. Treatment of anterior dental crossbite using bonded resin-composite slopes: case reports. Eur J Dent. 2008;2(4):303-6.

[36] Yaseen SM, Acharya R. Hexa Helix:Modified Quad Helix Appliance to Correct Anterior and Posterior Crossbites in Mixed Dentition. Case Reports in Dentistry. 2012: 1-5.

[37] Wiedel AP1, Bondemark L. Stability of anterior crossbite correction: A randomized controlled trial with a 2-year follow-up. Angle Orthod. 2014 Jul 8. [Epub ahead of print]

[38] Sanin C, Sekiguchi T, Savara BS. A clinical method for the prediction of closure of the central diastema. ASDC J Dent Child 1969; 36: 415–418.

[39] Baum AT. The midline diastema. J Oral Med 1966; 21: 30–39.

[40] Nainar SM, Gnanasundaram N. Incidence and etiology of midlinediastema in a population in southIndia (Madras). Angle Orthod 1989; 59: 277–282.

[41] Angle EH. Treatment of Malocclusion of the Teeth 7th edn. Philadelphia: SS White Dental Manufacturing Company, 1907: p167.

[42] Sicher H. Oral Anatomy 2nd edn. St Louis: CV Mosby Co, 1952: pp272–273.

[43] Edwards JG. The diastema, the frenum, the frenectomy: a clinical study. Am J Orthod 1977; 71:489–508.

[44] Popovich F, Thompson GW, Main PA. Persisting maxillary diastema: indications for treatment. Am JOrthod 1979; 75(4): 399–404.

[45] Proffit WR, Fields HW. Contemporary Orthodontics 2nd edn. St Louis: Mosby Yearbook, 1993: p467

[46] Shashua D, Artun J. Relapse afterorthodontic correction of maxillarymedian diastema: a follow-up evaluation of consecutive cases. Angle Orthod 1999; 69: 257–263.

[47] Nagalakshmi S, Sathish R, Priya K, Dhayanithi D. Changes in quality of life during orthodontic correction of midline diastema. J Pharm Bioallied Sci. 2014 (Suppl 1): 162-4

[48] Almeida RR, Almeida MR, Oltramari-Navarro PV, Conti AC, Navarro Rde L, Souza KR. Serial extraction: 20 years of follow-up. J Appl Oral Sci. 2012; 20(4):486-92.

[49] Hotz P.R. Guidance of eruption versus serial extraction. Am. J. Orthod, 1970; 58(1): 1-20.

[50] Nagalakshmi S, Sathish R, Priya K, Dhayanithi D. Changes in quality of life during orthodontic correction of midline diastema. J Pharm Bioallied Sci. 2014; 6 (Suppl 1):. [Epub ahead of print]

[51] Lee KP. The fallacy of serial extractions. Aust Orthod J. 2013;29(2):217-21.

[52] Almeida RR, Almeida MR, Oltramari-Navarro PV, Conti AC, Navarro Rde L, Souza KR. Serial extraction: 20 years of follow-up. J Appl Oral Sci. 2012 Jul-Aug;20(4): 486-92.

[53] Baume, L. J. Cephalo-facial growth patterns and the functional adaptation of the temporo-mandibular joint structures. Eur Orthod Soc Trans, 1969: 79—98.

[54] Calvert, F. J. () An assessment of Andresen therapy on Class II Division I malocclusion. Br J Orthodk 1982; 9: 149-153.

[55] Hamilton, S. D., Sinclair, P. M. & Hamilton, R. H. A cephalometric, tomographic and dental cast evaluation of Frankei therapy. Am J Orthod. 1987; 92: 427-434.

[56] Pancherz H. A cephalometric analysis of skeletal and dental changes contributing to Class II correction in activator treatment. Am J Orthod 1984;85:125-134

[57] Mills C, McCulloch K. Treatment effects of the Twin-block appliance: a cephalometric study. Am J Orthod 1998;114:15-24.

[58] Windmiller EC. Acrylic splint Herbst appliance: cephalometric evaluation. Am J Orthod Dentofac Orthop 1993;104:73-84.

[59] Baccetti T. et al. Treatment timing for Twin-block therapy. Am J Orthod dentofacial Orhop 2000;118:159-70.

[60] Usumez S, Uysal T, Sari Z, Basciftci FA, Karaman AI, Guray E. The effects of early preorthodontic trainer treatment on Class II, division 1 patients. Angle Orthod. 2004 Oct;74(5):605-9.

[61] Uysal T1, Yagci A, Kara S, Okkesim S. Influence of pre-orthodontic trainer treatment on the perioral and masticatory muscles in patients with Class II division 1 malocclusion. Eur J Orthod. 2012 34(1):96-101

[62] Hanoun AB, Khamis MF Mokhtar N. The effectiveness of the prefabricated myofunctional appliance T4FTM in comparison with Twin Block (TB) appliance in the treatment of Class II Div.1 malocclusion. A randomized clinical trial. Master thesis. School of Dental Sciences, University Science Malaysia, 2014.

3

Does the Demographic Transition Impact Health? The Oral Epidemiological Profile of the Elder Population

Javier de la Fuente Hernández,
Sergio Sánchez García,
Fátima del Carmen Aguilar Díaz,
Erika Heredia Ponce and
María del Carmen Villanueva Vilchis

1. Introduction

The term "demographic transition" was introduced more than 70 years ago to refer the process of changing from a traditional demographic model identified with high levels of mortality and birthrate to another one characterized by a fall on these indicators.

Between these conditions two phases can be identified: during the first one the growth rate of the population increases like a consequence of the decrease of the mortality, and during the second phase a deceleration of the population growth can be observed because of the decrease of fertility. Among the causes of this change of profile in the population we can find the process of industrialization, economic modernization, urbanization and the social and cultural changes.

The increase on life expectancy and the exposition to unhealthy lifestyles have modified the main causes of the morbidity and mortality, increasing the prevalence of non transmissible diseases. The first causes of mortality now fall in chronic degenerative diseases like diabetes *mellitus,* cardiovascular diseases or respiratory diseases. This change has been reflected as well in the oral status, determined by the life course of the individuals and the exposition to different risk factors. Through this chapter some of the oral conditions on elderly will be analyzed as well as the relationship between oral status and quality of life.

2. The demographic and epidemiologic transition

2.1. Demographic trends of the aging population — The international perspective

One of the best indicators of the improvement of the health of a population is ageing which is an intrinsic process of the demographic transition. The decline of the birthrate and the progressive rise of the life expectancy impact directly on the composition of the age groups of the population, reducing the number of persons in the younger age groups and expanding the segment of more advanced age groups.

The birthrate and mortality of the world population have decreased considerably particularly during the second half of the last century. The birthrate decreased between 1950-1955 and 2005-2010 from 37.0 to 20.0 births per 1000 persons [1]; while the mortality changed from 19.1 deaths per 1000 persons to 8.1 during the same period[2]. This transformation is known as demographic transition and has provoked a progressive increase of the size of the world population as well as its aging.

Migration can also affect aging in different ways, for example massive emigration due to circumstances like getting a better job, improving quality of life, or other motivations can reduce the number of young people, which can increase the ageing population [3].

The proportion of the world population over 60 years of age, of the most developed countries, will be increasing 1% per year before 2050 and it is expected to have increased 45% by mid-century, going from 287 millions in 2013 to 417 millions in 2050. In other words, 8% of the current population is 60 years old or more, but this proportion will be duplicated by 2050, reaching 19% that year[4].

The increase in life expectancy of the general population and particularly of the elderly around the world, should be considered like a success for humanity. The advance in preventive and curative technology of many diseases, coupled with the low exposure to risky conditions, increases the expectation to reach the elderly in better health conditions to live an adequate old age [3]. The increase in the life expectancy of the population poses a major challenge for public health, especially when we are going through a period in which poverty persists in those countries facing developing problems generating a bigger pressure on the already burdened health systems.

Aging is a continuous universal and irreversible process that can lead to a progressive lost of the ability to adapt. In healthy old individuals, many physiological functions are maintained, but when they are placed under stress, a loss of the functional reserve is revealed.

Aging is not a condition that is necessarily associated with disease and dependency, but it is a fact that the accumulative effect of multiple exposures and the unfavorable psychological, physical and social conditions increase the risk of older people to get sick [5]. It starts during the early years of the adult life, but it manifests some decades later, when people are called old. One unfair way to define elderness is to affirm that it starts with the age of retirement (60 or 65), but physiologically individuals get older in a different rate and some persons live more than 80 years. In developed countries, a person is considered old when he/she reaches the age of 65 years or more, but in developing countries 60 is considered as the starting point [6]

The countries with a more advanced stage of demographic transition recognize the need to evaluate the models for provision of health services for the elderly and achieve the mainte-nance of the pension systems and sanitary assistance despite all the requirements of the fast growing segment of older people in the population. However, the difficulties in the attention of the sanitary, social and economical needs may vary considerably by region. A common principle for the action is the need to focus on health promotion and the reduction of the dependency of elders.

Daily, seniors face risk situations that threaten their integrity and can alter the functions and structures of their body, if this happens, they face their environment in a different way and frequently the environmental and personal factors can force them to limit their activities. Therefore the functioning or disability of the individual must be seen as the result of the interaction between the health condition and the environment. Although different geographic, social or economical factors contribute to the functional dependency of seniors, chronic diseases are one of the main factors that impact this functioning and can even be its direct cause; this has been demonstrated in some previous studies in different populations. [7,8,9]

The aging process can affect the individual and social development, as well as the relative well-being of the younger persons. Among the factors with the greatest repercussion are the pension and retirement systems, the active population and its participation, the arrangements with the family and home, the intra-family transfers from one generation to other and the health condition of seniors. The importance of each one of these aspects can vary and depends of the demographic regimens and the institutional idiosyncrasy of every country. All countries in different levels and in different moments will have to include the topic of the repercussion of aging of the population in their priority issues on the health public and economic field.

3. Oral health problems in the elder population

The analysis of the oral health of elders has taken interest recently due to the accelerated changes on the demographic structure. Old people have poorer oral health, they seek oral health services less, and lose more teeth due to chronic conditions, they represent an important part of the health budget. [11, 12, 13].

The knowledge of the main problems of oral health of this population, is valuable in the planning of effective strategies that optimize the programs and has a positive effect in oral and general health. Among the main problems that affect the oral health there are:

3.1. Disorders of the oral mucosa

In the oral mucosa of old people there may be atrophy of the epithelium, decrease of the keratin and number of cells of the connective tissue, an increase of the intercellular substance and decrease in the oxygen consume. When there is a lack of elasticity of the mucosa with dryness and atrophy, hyperkeratosis can be found. The oral mucosa can present changes related to local factors that are acquired through the course of life like malnutrition, systemic diseases, the use of pharmacological drugs, unhealthy habits and others that can cause the thinning of the mucosa, making it smooth, dry and more permeable to harmful substances. Oral squamous cell carcinoma and pemphigoid carcinoma are almost exclusive of the elderly. [14,15]

3.2. Tooth loss

Complete or partial prosthesis is the most common treatment for tooth loss. Tooth loss has a deep emotional meaning; it symbolically reveals ageing and weakness. It is important to point out that in developing countries the oral care for the elderly has focused on dental extraction, and is the principal cause of the low number of remaining teeth. [16, 17]

Although the number of persons keeping their natural dentition has grown considerably during the last decades, the mean number of remaining teeth may vary according to the school level and the income. Thus it is pertinent to study tooth loss like a social issue according to the social determinants of health, since individuals with lowest school levels tend to a major loss of teeth [18].

3.3. Conditions related to the use of dentures

Denture stomatitis is one of the most frequent diseases that affect the oral tissues in denture wearers. [19] The prevalence of denture stomatitis is from 11 to 67% [20] and there are some factors involved like:

3.3.1. Hygiene of the prosthesis

The prevalence of denture stomatitis has been strongly correlated with hygiene [21,22]. The surface of the prosthesis can be a reservoir for plaque that conforms an ecosystem with a particular pH that can be influenced by the diet, saliva and other factors [23].

3.3.2. Prosthetic trauma

This is caused by maladjusted prosthetic devices and bad habits in their use [19, 20].

3.3.3. Candidiasis infection

The presence of plaque promotes the colonization of fungi species like candida on the prosthetic surface or the mucosa [19,20,22]. The Candida fungi, mainly the genre *Albicans* is a part of the normal flora of the oral cavity, but in some circumstances it is able to develop and produce infection, although some authors mention that there are other involved species [24, 25].

The typical lesions of oral candidiasis are white plaques that are easy to remove on the oral, oropharyngeal and palatal mucosa; in some cases there is angular cheilitis as well. The predisposing factors are xerostomy, treatment with broad-spectrum antibiotics, the use of inhaled corticosteroids and alterations of the cellular immunity [25,26].

When candidiasis infection is associated with old removable prosthetics or maladjusted devices, it can induce the formation of denture stomatitis [27,28]. The treatment for the condition is the eradication of the local factors and therefore the prosthetic devices must be removed a long period, good hygiene conditions should be kept as well as using mouth rinses and antifungal medication.

3.4. Dietetic factors

The diet of the elderly is characterized for being very limited since the lack of a denture in good conditions avoids eating fresh fruits and vegetables or raw food. The diet is regularly is composed of canned food, which can cause vitamin deficiencies and therefore hematological deficit [29]

3.5. Caries

Caries can be considered an infectious disease caused by multiple factors: biologic, social, economical, cultural and environmental. Its formation and development is conditioned by the lifestyle of the individual. It affects the crown and root of the teeth and in the absence of dental attention it can cause the loss of the tooth and it constitutes a source of infection for the organism.

This disease occurs on the dental structures in contact with the microbial deposits (biofilm) and due to the imbalance between the tooth substance and the plaque surrounding fluid, there is a loss of minerals on the dental surface which leads to located destruction of the hard tissues.

The prevalence of dental caries in developed countries has decreased because a high sector of the old population has access to dental services promoting a major use of dental prevention measures, this allows, that the individuals keep a higher number of functional teeth [18,30]

The other kind of caries, root caries, is very common in the elderly since it is a consequence of the gingival recession. The root surface, composed by cementum and dentin is more suscep-tible to the oral environment than the crown surface composed by enamel and dentin [31,32]

The reported prevalence of root caries is from 24 to 37% in some populations [33]. Almost all the published studies reporting incidence have included old people from public institutions, patients with periodontal disease, participants of some clinic studies and some communities, however they have reported to 10 to 40% incidence [32,34].

Loss of periodontal attachment, low salivary flow, presence of caries in the past, cognitive impairment, use of some kind of medication, low scholar level, high number of cariogenic microorganisms, and the lack of dental attention are among the most studied risk factors for root caries [35].

3.6. Periodontal disease

Periodontal disease constitutes one of the main causes of tooth loss [16]. Traditionally it was accepted that the loss of epithelial attachment and alveolar bone was caused by the periodontal changes related to the ageing process, however nowadays the theory indicates that is not like that.

The periodontum reacts to ageing in two ways: if there is low hygiene, the plaque accumulation affects the periodontal tissues causing gingivitis and in some susceptible patients the retraction of the gingival tissue, formation of gingival pockets and dental loss. However in some old patients there can be tissue recovery with a minimal change on the marginal gingival, narrowness of the periodontal ligament, firm adherence of the teeth, and accumulation of cementum [14,36]

3.7. Xerostomy or low salivary flow

Saliva is a complex exocrine secretion, important for the maintenance of the homeostasis of the oral cavity. The salivary functions in relation with the flow and molecular composition (proteins, glycoproteins and phosphoproteins) are well known: the protection of the oral tissues against desiccation and the environmental attacks, the modulation of the desmineral-ization-remineralization processes, the lubrication of the occlusal surfaces and the mainte-nance of the ecological balance [37].

The protection of the salivary flow in the elderly can be reduce because of the medical prescription of some drugs for the treatment of certain conditions in this age group like depression or other systemic conditions like hypertension [38,39].

Although it has not been well demonstrated, a physiological decrease of the salivary flow may occur with aging, however it seems that structural alterations may occur in some salivary glands, concretely submandibular and minor glands, however, despite all these conditions the global functioning and the salivary volume is not modified.

The cause of the xerostomy or the decrease on the salivary flow is more related to the existence of some diseases like hypertension, diabetes *mellitus*, Sjögren syndrome, rheumatoid condi-tions, cystic fibrosis, neurological conditions, depression and immune system dysfunction and their treatment, since most of them have a repercussion on the salivary glands [40,41].

3.8. Oral cancer

This disease is related with aging, since nearly 95% of the cases take place in people 40 years of age and older and the mean age of the diagnosis is around 60. It is estimated that half of the cases of cancer are in people 65 years of age. [42,43,44].

The etiology of oral cancer and precancerous lesions is multiple. The most common cited factors are: tobacco and alcohol consumption, genetics, nutrition, the presence of some virus, radiations and occupational risks in addition to use of maladjusted dental prostheses, de-stroyed teeth by caries or trauma and low oral hygiene.

Most of these factors have an accumulative effect with time, and due to this effect, many authors affirm that age is the main risk factor for the development of oral cancer [44,45]. The early detection of the malignant lesions is fundamental for providing the best prognosis of this disease.

3.9. Pain

Pain is often a manifestation of the oral problems reflected on other facial structures like the orbital frontal region that can be confounded with classic headache.

Sometimes, pain appears like a consequence of the degenerative phenomena of the structures that support the oral cavity (bones, joints muscles and others). Among these phenomena we can find osteoarthritis and osteoporosis of the jaw, or disorders on the temporomandibular jaw that can cause pain, snaps and the added locking of joint function like limitation to the mouth opening and difficulty for chewing [46].

The temporomandibular dysfunction is frequent in old people and it is characterized by constant pain on the periauricular area, otic pain that can increase while the patient is chewing, or in patients with bruxism, when they clench teeth consciously or unconsciously during stress [47,48].

4. Links between oral health and systemic diseases

It is clear that oral health problems affect the general condition of old people. Many systemic diseases have specific signs in the mouth that allow the diagnosis. Among them we can find genetic diseases, systemic infections, immune alterations, neoplasms, nutritional problems, connective tissue diseases, gastrointestinal diseases, renal diseases, cardiovascular diseases, endocrine diseases, dermatologic diseases, neurologic diseases and skeletal diseases. There are also some medications that can affect the consistency and characteristics of the saliva and that can alter the texture of the tongue, or affect the gingiva [36,37,48,49,50]

4.1. Periodontal disease related to systemic diseases

Among the conditions related to periodontal disease and the cardiovascular system we can find bacterial endocarditis, myocardial infarction, ischemic heart disease, thrombosis, coronary heart disease and varicose veins [51].

The links between periodontal disease and respiratory diseases can be established only if the defensive mechanisms fail. The most commonly associated conditions are the bacterial pneumonia, bronchitis, chronic obstructive pulmonary disease and lung abscesses [52,53,54].

The bacteria create their own ecological niches on different surfaces of the mouth like teeth, gingival sulcus, dorsal area of the tongue and oral and pharyngeal mucosa using the saliva and crevicular fluid like their main nutritional source, and through bacteremia, derive in systemic processes. The sepsis is the responsible for the beginning and progression of diverse inflammatory diseases like arthritis, peptic ulcers and appendicitis [54]

Pneumonia is the infection of the lung parenchyma caused by several infectious agents that include bacteria, fungi, parasites and viruses. Bacteria of the oral flora like *Actinobacillus actinomycetem-commitans, Actinomyces Israeli,* and the anaerobic *P gingivalis,* and *Fusobacteri-*

um, can be aspirated and taken to the lower airways and cause pneumonia [55,56]. The source can be from bacteria of the normal flora or from periodontal cases [56].

5. Oral health related quality of life in the elder population

The relationship between quality of life and oral health has been understood like a multidimensional concept that reports the aspects concerning to oral health including the functional, social and pshycological aspect of the individuals [57,58,59,60].

One of the major contributions of dentistry is to improve and maintain the quality of life of the person since most oral diseases and their consequences have an impact on the performance of daily activities [36].

The contemporary concepts of health suggest that oral health could be defined as the physical, psychological and social wellbeing in relation to the dental status as well as the hard and soft tissues of the oral cavity and not only absence of disease [36]. This definition proposes that the measure of oral health not only has to take into account oral indexes that measure the presence or severity of a pathology (physical well-being) but it must also complemented with social and pshycological measures [36,60,61].

Traditionally, the methods used to estimate oral health, have been limited to clinic indicators or oral indexes, and the presence or absence of disease. This view leaves out all the subjective measures, in other words the perception of the persons about their oral health status.

This view about oral health related quality of life (OHRQOL) promotes the knowledge of the origin and behavior of the oral diseases, largely because the social factors and the environment are the main causes of these diseases and some interventions can be applied [62,63,64]).

In elder people, the self-perception of oral health can be affected by the perception of other personal values, like the belief that some pains and disabilities are unavoidable because of the ageing. These ideas can lead to the over and under estimation of the oral health condition. The available information about self-perception is subjective, and for this reason the perception about how oral health affects the quality of life must be evaluated according to instruments that have been adapted and validated on specific populations.

The dental status in old people has a repercussion on their ability to perform daily activities affecting their quality of life with a bigger impact on some activities such as eating, speaking and pronunciation [61]

The existing subjective measures on oral health as well as the focus on oral health cannot provide data that helps the decision makers to allocate the resources related with improving the oral health of the elderly, however they can give an idea about the degree of affection for the individual and populations [62].

6. Conclusions

Oral health problems among old people are caused mainly by the accumulation of sequels that the null assistance to the dental services has left as well as the lack of self-care in this age group.

The most common affections are the tooth loss, coronal and root caries, periodontal diseases, lesions derived from the use of defective prosthesis and temporomandibular joint pain. Besides, this group, can also present oral cancer and oral manifestations of other systemic diseases. These conditions are associated with pain when chewing, a frequent reason of consultation in primary care.

It is important to continue studying the convergence of sociodemographic information with the oral health diagnosis, to determine the therapeutic needs and the factors that make it difficult to access the dental services and to design adequate interventions to solve the most common oral health problems of this group of the population.

Public and private oral health services must prevent the onset of diseases that can produce serious effects on quality of life of the elderly.

Author details

Javier de la Fuente Hernández[1], Sergio Sánchez García[2,3], Fátima del Carmen Aguilar Díaz[1], Erika Heredia Ponce[3] and María del Carmen Villanueva Vilchis[1*]

*Address all correspondence to: vv.carmen@gmail.com

1 Escuela Nacional de Estudios Superiores, Unidad León. Universidad Nacional Autónoma de México, México

2 Unidad de Investigación en Epidemiología y Servicios de Salud. Área Envejecimiento. Centro Médico Nacional Siglo XXI. Instituto Mexicano del Seguro Social, México

3 Departamento de Salud Pública y Epidemiología Bucal. Facultad de Odontología. Universidad Nacional Autónoma de México, México

References

[1] United Nations, Department of Economic and Social Affairs. Worls Population Prospects: The 2012 Revision; Excel tables-Fertility Data "Crude Birth Rate". Available en: http://esa.un.org/wpp/Excel-Data/fertility.htm

[2]   United Nations, Department of Economic and Social Affairs. Worls Population Prospects: The 2012 Revision; Excel tables-Mortality Data "Crude Death Rate". Available en: http://esa.un.org/wpp/excel-data/mortality.htm

[3]   United Nations, Department of Economic and Social Affairs, Population Division (2013). World Population Ageing 2013. ST/ESA/SER.A/348.

[4]   World Population Prospects: The 2012 Revision. Key Findings and Advance Tables. United Nations Department of Economic and Social Affairs/Population Division, Working Paper No. ESA/P/WP.227, June 13, 2013, 54 p.

[5]   Gutiérrez Robledo LM, García Peña MC, Jiménez Bolón JE. Envejecimiento y dependencia. Realidades y previsión para los próximos años. México: Intersistemas Editores, 2014.

[6]   Organización Panamericana de la Salud. Salud en las personas de edad. Envejecimiento y salud: un cambio de paradigma. E.U., Washington D.C., 1998.

[7]   Sousa RM, Ferri CP, Acosta D, Guerra M, Huang Y, Jacob K, Jotheeswaran A, Hernandez MA, Liu Z, Pichardo GR, Rodriguez JJ, Salas A, Sosa AL, Williams J, Zuniga T, Prince M. The contribution of chronic diseases to the prevalence of dependence among older people in Latin America, China and India: a 10/66 Dementia Research Group population-based survey. BMC Geriatr. 2010;10:53.

[8]   Daigo Yoshida, Toshiharu Ninomiya, Yasufumi Doi, Jun Hata, Masayo Fukuhara, Fumie Ikeda, Naoko Mukai, Yutaka Kiyohara. Prevalence and Causes of Functional Disability in an Elderly General Population of Japanese: The Hisayama Study. J Epidemiol. 2012; 22:222–229

[9]   Wolff JL, Boult C, Boyd C, Anderson G. Newly reported chronic conditions and onset of functional dependency. J Am Geriatr Soc. 2005;53:851-5.

[10] Kalache, A. y Coombes, Y. Population aging and care of the elderly in Latin America and the Caribbean. Review of Clinical Gerontology, 1995; 5:347-355.

[11] Medina-Solís CE, Pérez-Núñez R, Maupomé G, Avila-Burgos L, Pontigo-Loyola AP, Patiño-Marín N, Villalobos-Rodelo JJ. National survey on edentulism and its geographic distribution, among Mexicans 18 years of age and older (with emphasis in WHO age groups). J Oral Rehabil 2008;35:237-244.

[12] Marino R. Oral health of the elderly: reality, myth, and perspective. Bull Pan Am Health Organ 1994;28:202-210.

[13] Sánchez-García S, Heredia-Ponce E, Cruz-Hervert P, Juárez-Cedillo T, Cárdenas-Bahena A, García-Peña C. Oral health status in older adults with social security in Mexico City: latent class analysis. J Clin Exp Dent. 2014;6(1):e29-35.

[14] Mckenna G, Burke FM. Age-related oral changes. Dent Update. 2010 Oct;37(8): 519-23.

[15] Silverman S Jr. Mucosal lesions in older adults. J Am Dent Assoc. 2007 Sep;138 Suppl:41S-46S.

[16] Renvert S, Persson RE, Persson GR. Tooth loss and periodontitis in older individuals: results from the Swedish National Study on Aging and Care. J Periodontol. 2013 Aug;84(8):1134-44.

[17] Dable RA, Yashwante BJ, Marathe SS, Gaikwad BS, Patil PB, Momin AA. Tooth loss--how emotional it is for the elderly in India? Oral Health Dent Manag. 2014 Jun;13(2): 305-10.

[18] Slade GD, Akinkugbe AA, Sanders AE. Projections of U.S. Edentulism Prevalence Following 5 Decades of Decline. J Dent Res. 2014 Aug 21. pii: 0022034514546165. [Epub ahead of print]

[19] Wilson J. The aetiology, diagnosis and management of denture stomatitis. Br Dent J. 1998 Oct 24;185(8):380-384.

[20] Jeganathan S, Lin CC. Denture stomatitis--a review of the aetiology, diagnosis and management. Aust Dent J. 1992 Apr;37(2):107-14.

[21] Vigild M. Oral mucosal lesions among institutionalized elderly in Denmark. Community Dent Oral Epidemiol, 1987; 15:309-313.

[22] Salerno C, Pascale M, Contaldo M, Esposito V, Busciolano M, Milillo L, Guida A, Petruzzi M, Serpico R. Candida-associated denture stomatitis. Med Oral Patol Oral Cir Bucal. 2011 Mar 1;16(2):e139-43.

[23] Catalan A, Herrera R, Martinez A. Denture plaque and palatal mucosa in denture stomatitis: scanning electron microscopic and microbiologic study. J Prosthet Dent. 1987 May;57(5):581-6.

[24] Morimoto K, Kihara A, Suetsugu T. Clinico-pathological study on denture stomatitis. J Oral Rehabil. 1987

[25] Guinea J. Global trends in the distribution of Candida species causing candidemia. Clin Microbiol Infect. 2014 Jun;20 Suppl 6:5-10.

[26] Kulak-Ozkan Y, Kazazoglu E, Arikan A. Oral hygiene habits, denture cleanliness, presence of yeasts and stomatitis in elderly people. J Oral Rehabil, 2002; 29:300-304.

[27] Marinoski J, Bokor-Bratić M, Canković M. Is denture stomatitis always related with candida infection? A case control study. Med Glas (Zenica). 2014 Aug;11(2):379-84.

[28] Peltola MK1, Raustia AM, Salonen MA. Effect of complete denture renewal on oral health--a survey of 42 patients. J Oral Rehabil. 1997 Jun;24(6):419-25.

[29] García-Arias MT, Villarino Rodríguez A, García-Linares MC, Rocandio AM, García-Fernández MC. Iron, folate and vitamins B12 & C dietary intake of an elderly institutionalized population in León, Spain. Nutr Hosp. 2003 Jul-Aug;18(4):222-5.

[30] Glass RL. The first international conference on the declining prevalence of dental caries Secular changes in caries prevalence in two Massachusetts towns. J Dent Res,
1982; 61 (Spec Issue):1301-1383.

[31] Papapanou PN, Wennström JL, Gröndahl K. Periodontal status in relation to age and
tooth type. A cross-sectional radiographic study. J Clin Periodontol. 1988 Aug;15(7):
469-78.

[32] Bignozzi I, Crea A, Capri D, Littarru C, Lajolo C, Tatakis DN. Root caries: a periodontal perspective. J Periodontal Res. 2014 Apr;49(2):143-63. doi: 10.1111/jre.12094.
Epub 2013 May 7.

[33] Beck, J. D. Indentification of risk factors. In: Bader, J. D., USA: ed. Risk assessment in
dentistry. Chapel Hill, University of North Carolina Dental Ecology, 1990.

[34] Sánchez-García S, Reyes-Morales H, Juárez-Cedillo T, Espinel-Bermúdez C, Solórzano-Santos F, García-Peña C. A prediction model for root caries in an elderly population. Community Dentistry and Oral Epidemiology 2011 Feb;39(1):44-52.

[35] Saunders RH Jr, Meyerowitz C. Dental caries in older adults. Dent Clin North Am
2005; 49:293-308.

[36] Sánchez-García S, Juárez-Cedillo T, Heredia-Ponce E, García-Peña C. El envejecimiento de la población y la Salud Bucodental. Breviarios de Seguridad Social. México
D.F.: Centro Interamericano de Estudios de Seguridad Social, Edito; 2013. ISBN:
978-607-8088-14-0.

[37] Sreebny LM. Saliva in health and disease: an appraisal and update. Int Dent J. 2000
Jun;50(3):140-61.

[38] Närhi TO, Vehkalahti MM, Siukosaari P, Ainamo A. Salivary findings, daily medication and root caries in the old elderly. Caries Res. 1998;32(1):5-9.

[39] Gerdin EW, Einarson S, Jonsson M, Aronsson K, Johansson I. Impact of dry mouth
conditions on oral health-related quality of life in older people. Gerodontology. 2005
Dec;22(4):219-26.

[40] Sreebny L. Saliva: its role in health and disease. Int Dent J 1992; 42: 291–304.

[41] Sánchez-García S, Gutiérrez-Venegas G, Juárez-Cedillo T, Reyes-Morales H, Solórzano-Santos F, García-Peña C. A simplified caries risk bacteriologic test in stimulated
saliva from elderly patients. Gerodontology 2008; 25: 26-33.

[42] Silverman S. Oral cancer. 3ªed. EUA, Atlanta: American Cancer Society, 1990.

[43] Canto MT, Devesa SS. Oral cavity and pharynx cancer incidence rates in the United
States, 1975-1998. Oral Oncol. 2002 Sep;38(6):610-7.

[44] Sánchez-García S, Juárez Cedillo T, Espinel Bermudez MC, Mould Quevedo JF, Gó-
mez Dantés H, de La Fuente Hernández J, Leyva Huerta ER, García Peña C. Egresos

Hospitalarios por cáncer bucal en el Instituto Mexicano del Seguro Social, 1991-2000. Rev Med Inst Mex Seguro Soc 2008; 46 (1): 101-108.

[45]   Hunter KD, Yeoman CM. An update on the clinical pathology of oral precancer and cancer. Dent Update. 2013 Mar;40(2):120-2, 125-6.

[46]   Serrano Garijo, P. y otros. La salud bucodental en los mayores. Prevención y cuidados para una prevención integral. En: Promoción de salud en los mayores, volumen 6. Madrid, Instituto de Salud Pública, 2003.

[47]   Sánchez-García S, Heredia-Ponce E, Villanueva Vilchis M del C, Rabay Gánem C. Dolor para masticar. En García Peña M del C, Gutiérrez Robledo LM, Arango Lopera VE, Pérez-Zepeda MU. Geriatría para el médico familiar. Manual Moderno. Edito; 2012.

[48]   Smith BJ, Valdez IH, Berkey DB. Oral problems. En: Ham RJ, Sloane PD, Warshaw GA, Bernard MA, Flaherty E. Primary care geriatrics: a case-based approach. 5th ed Mosby, 2007.

[49]   Mariño R, Albala C, Sanchez H, Cea X, Fuentes A. Prevalence of Diseases and Conditions Which Impact on Oral Health and Oral Health Self-Care Among Older Chilean. J Aging Health. 2014 May 21.

[50]   Gaffen SL, Herzberg MC, Taubman MA, Van Dyke TE. Recent advances in host defense mechanisms/therapies against oral infectious diseases and consequences for systemic disease. Adv Dent Res. 2014 May;26(1):30-7.

[51]   Demmer RT, Kocher T, Schwahn C, Völzke H, Jacobs DR Jr, Desvarieux M. Refining exposure definitions for studies of periodontal disease and systemic disease associations. Community Dent Oral Epidemiol. 2008 Dec;36(6):493-502. doi: 10.1111/j. 1600-0528.2008.00435.x. Epub 2008 Apr 14.

[52]   Papapanou Panos, N. Populations studies of microbial ecology periodontal health and diseases. Ann Periodontol 2003; 7:54-61.

[53]   Bansal M, Rastogi S, Vineeth NS. Influence of periodontal disease on systemic disease: inversion of a paradigm: a review. J Med Life. 2013 Jun 15;6(2):126-30.

[54]   Scannapieco, F. A. Position paper: periodontal disease as a potential risk factor for systemic diseases. J. Periodontol, 1998; 69:841-850.

[55]   Reynolds MA. Modifiable risk factors in periodontitis: at the intersection of aging and disease. Periodontol 2000. 2014 Feb;64(1):7-19.

[56]   Scannapieco, F. A., Papandonatos, G. y otros. Associations between oral conditions and respiratory disease in a national sample survey population. Ann. Periodontol, 1998; 3:251-256.

[57]   Cohen, K. y Jago, J. D. Toward the formulation of socio-dental indicators. Int J Health Serv, 1976; 6:681-687.

[58] WHO definition of health. Fecha de consulta: 1 de septiembre de 2014: URL: www.who.int/about/definition/en/print.html.

[59] Engel, G. L. The clinical application of biopsychosocial model. Am J Psychiatry, 1980; 137:535-544.

[60] Sánchez-García S, Heredia-Ponce E, Juárez-Cedillo T, Gallegos-Carrillo K, Espinel-Bermúdez C, De la Fuente-Hernández J, García-Peña C. Psychometric properties of the General Oral Health Assessment Index (GOHAI) and their relationship in the state of dentition of an elderly Mexican population. Journal of Public Health Dentistry 2010;70(4):300-307.

[61] Sánchez-García S, Juárez-Cedillo T, Reyes-Morales H, De la Fuente-Hernández J, Solórzano-Santos F, García-Peña C. Estado de la dentición y sus efectos en la capacidad de los ancianos para desempeñar sus actividades habituales. Salud Pública Mex 2007;49 (3): 173-181.

[62] Petersen PE, Kandelman D, Arpin S, Ogawa H. Global oral health of older people–call for public health action. Community Dent Health 2010;27:257–267.

[63] Cushing, A. M., Sheiham, A. y otros. Developing socio-dental indicators – the social impact of dental disease. Community Dental Health 1986; 3:3-17.

[64] Locker, D. Measuring oral health: A conceptual framework. Community Dent Health, 1988; 5:3-18.

4

Oral Health From Dental Paleopathology

Hisashi Fujita

1. Introduction

Since when have humans been afflicted with dental diseases? It is not easy to find an answer to this question. There are two main methods to examine what types of disease our ancestors suffered. One method involves the history of medicine or a study called "medical history," which mainly examines pathologies written in ancient documents and ancient writings and attempts to identify the diseases. Michinaga Fujiwara was a powerful individual in the Heian period of Japan (794-1192 AD) [1]. He was speculated to have died of complications of diabetes based on the records of his pathology in the literature. This type of finding is the result of research in the history of medicine (a study of medical history). The other method involves a field of study in physical anthropology called "paleopathology," in which the author of this paper specializes. In paleopathology, the research materials are hard tissues such as bones and teeth from humans of ancient times and obtained from archeological excavations (needless to say, the soft tissues have long decomposed and returned to soil). Thus, it is possible to learn about the frequency of certain diseases in the past in groups of people and about the true pathology at the time of death. In this paper, a few dental diseases were interpreted from the perspective of an anthropologist who handles ancient human skeletal remains. These diseases can be indicators of modern oral health.

2. Two major diseases in the oral cavity are caries and periodontal disease

This statement is believed to have been true since the ancient times. In a previous study, the author of this paper described that, before the introduction of modern dentistry, people were more affected by caries and periodontal disease, the main cause of tooth loss, because they were unable to receive scientific dental care. Modern humans can obtain nutrients parenterally and via gastrostomy with the advancement of modern medicine. For the majority of human history, the mouth was the only means through which people have taken in nutrients. Therefore, tooth loss was speculated to have caused malnutrition and even death in many pre-modern individuals with numerous missing teeth. In the pre-modern times, longevity was likely dependent on the preservation of one's own teeth to obtain sufficient nutrients.

2.1. Tooth loss in human skeletal remains of Japan

Trinkaus reported on the problem of tooth loss in the La Chapelle-aux-Saints Neanderthal from approximately 60,000 years ago, the most ancient material that has been examined for this purpose [2]. He reported that 51.7% of the teeth were missing antemortem in this Nean-derthal. In another study, Trinkaus also reported that 25% of the teeth were missing in the Shanidar Neanderthals [3]. It is difficult to obtain a large sample size of ancient human fossils, and consequently adequate statistical analysis cannot be performed due to small sample size. Therefore, the information from these ancient human fossils is merely for reference.

There are some case reports worldwide on tooth loss in Homo sapiens [4-8], but the number of studies on ancient human skeletal remains is not large. These researchers, except the author of this paper, used all examined individuals as materials. Thus, a bias likely occurred regarding the types of teeth, which were sometimes located in areas of defects in ancient human skeletal remains. The author of this paper examined remaining teeth in ancient human skeletal remains excavated from archeological sites of the pre-modern periods in Japan: the Kofun period (3rd–early7th century), Kamakura period (1192–1333 AD), Muromachi period (1335–1573 AD), and Edo period (1603–1868 AD). A total of 329 individuals were examined, of whom 145 individuals were selected as materials because their sex was determinable and their maxillary and mandibular alveolar bones were fully examinable (Table 1). This material selection method enabled data collection without bias for all tooth types. The estimation of age and determination of sex were performed by morphological observations of anthropological bones. Since the number of materials was not large, the individuals of different sexes were pooled together. The individuals were divided into three groups: early middle age group (approximately 20-39 years), late middle age group (approximately 40-49 years), and old age group (50 years or older).

In this study, the ancient human skeletal remains used as materials were grouped by time period and by age group. Table 1 shows the number of individuals and the number of examinable teeth. In all time periods as shown in Table 2, there was a tendency for the number of missing teeth to increase with age, progressing from early middle age to late middle age to old age. In the Kofun period, the mean number of missing teeth was 2.67 (SD: 1.63) in early middle age, 6.00 (SD: 2.00) in late middle age, and 16.00 in old age. In the Kamakura period, the mean number was 1.17 (SD: 1.47), 2.22 (SD: 2.10), and 4.50 (SD: 2.12), respectively. In the Muromachi period, the mean number was 1.80 (SD: 0.84), 5.80 (SD: 4.55), and 21.00, respectively. In the Edo period, the mean number was 2.31 (SD: 2.58), 5.18 (SD: 4.57), and 29.67 (SD: 4.04), respectively. Table 3 shows whether there is a difference in the number of missing teeth by age group after combining all the materials of different time periods. The results revealed that the number of missing teeth differed significantly (p<0.01) between the early middle age and late middle age groups and between the late middle age and old age groups, statistically indicating increasing tooth loss with age in pre-modern Japanese people. Table 4 shows the number of missing teeth in the maxilla and mandible. The number of missing teeth is shown by time period and by age group, but there were many time periods without a sufficient number of materials. Therefore, the lower portion of the table shows the number of maxillary missing teeth and the number of mandibular missing teeth of all time periods. A significance test was used to determine the difference in the number of missing teeth between the maxilla and mandible, and there was no significant difference between the jaws in any age group. Figures 1 and 2 show the percentages of missing teeth of all tooth types in the maxilla and mandible, respectively. In general, the percentage of missing teeth tended to be lower in the anterior teeth and the percentage tended to be higher in the posterior teeth.

Period	Group	Number of individuals	Number of Observed teeth[a]
Kofun	Early middle age	6	192
	Late middle age	7	224
	Old age	1	32
Kamakura	Early middle age	18	576
	Late middle age	18	576
	Old age	2	64
Muromchi	Early middle age	5	160
	Late middle age	5	160
	Old age	1	32
Edo	Early middle age	45	1440
	Larly middle age	34	1088
	Old age	3	96
Total		145	4640

[a]The number of observed teeth includes ante-mortem tooth loss and post-mortem tooth loss.

Table 1. The archaeological materials used from Kofun, Kamakura, Muromachi and Edo periods in Japan.

Period	Group	Lost teeth	Observed teeth	Average of number of ante-mortem teeth per person	SD
Kofun	Early middle age	16	192	2.67	1.63
	Late middle age	42	224	6.00	2.00
	Old age	16	32	16.00	-
Kamakura	Early middle age	21	576	1.17	1.47
	Late middle age	40	576	2.22	2.10
	Old age	9	64	4.50	2.12

Period	Group	Lost teeth	Observed teeth	Average of number of ante-mortem teeth per person	SD
Muromachi	Early middle age	9	160	1.80	0.84
	Late middle age	29	160	5.80	4.55
	Old age	21	32	21.00	-
Edo[a]	Early middle age	104	1440	2.31	2.58
	Late middle age	176	1088	5.18	4.57
	Old age	89	96	29.67	4.04

[a]Data were cited from Fujita[18].

Table 2. The number of ante-mortem tooth loss by age distribution.

	Significant
Early middle age-Late middle age	***
Late middleage-Old age	***

***: $P < 0.001$

Table 3. Comparison of number of missing teeth by age distribution.

		Tooth type					
		Upper			Lower		
Early middle age	URM1	ULM1	Total	LRM1	LLM1	Total	Grand total
Observed	36	34	70	31	31	61	131
Average	3.13	3.24	3.19	2.16	2.27	2.23	2.74
SD	0.99	1.05	1.01	0.9	0.87	0.86	1.06
Early middle age vs Late middle age	P=0.165 ns	P=0.104 ns	P<0.05 L>E	P<0.05 L>E	P=0.218 ns	P<0.01 L>E	P<0.05 L>E
Late middle age	URM1	ULM1	Total	LRM1	LLM1	Total	Grand total
Observed	11	9	20	8	7	15	35
Average	3.91	3.89	3.9	3.13	2.71	2.93	3.49
SD	1.64	1.05	1.37	1.25	0.76	1.03	1.31

ns: not significance

E: Early middle age; L: Late middle age

Table 4. Alveoler resession of Somali people in Early middle age and Late middle age.

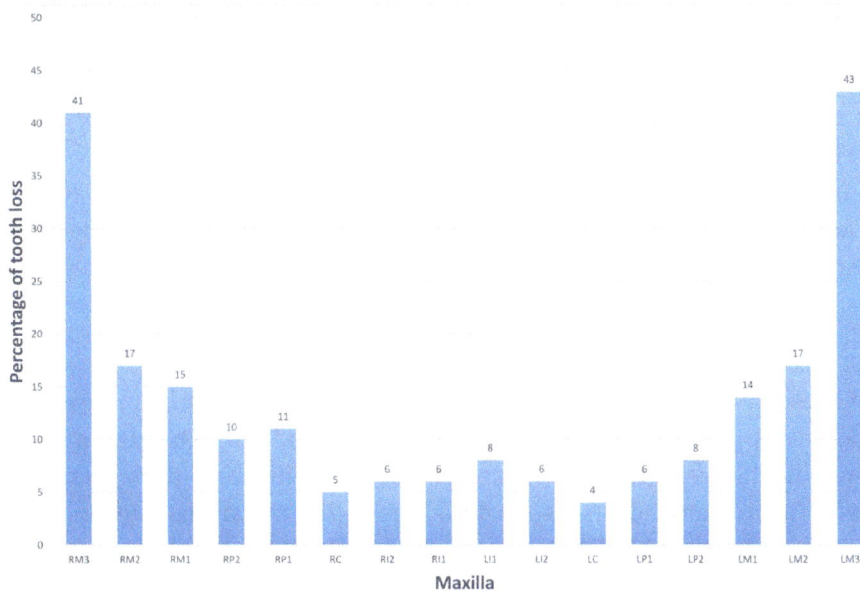

Figure 1. The rate of loss by tooth type in Maxilla in pre-modern periods in Japan.

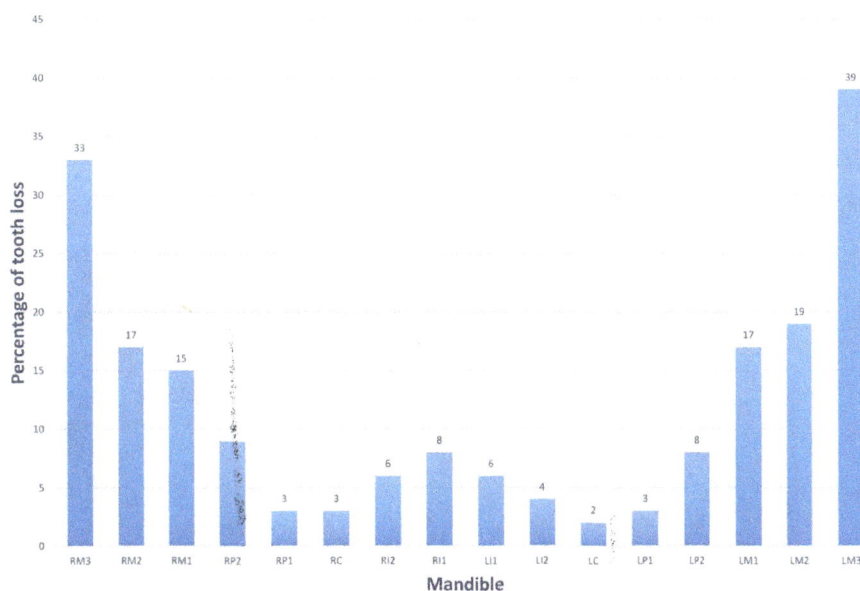

Figure 2. The rate of loss by tooth type in mandible in pre-modern periods in Japan.

In the early and late middle age individuals, the low number of missing teeth had been maintained at 1.11 to 6.00 teeth from the Kofun period to Edo period, spanning 1500 years. This result might be very surprising for health care providers as well as for the general public. The assumption is that people in olden times lost many teeth at an early age, but it is not consistent with the results of this study. At least to late middle age, the number of missing teeth was lower in pre-modern times than in modern time. Lopez *et al.* made a similar finding in a study comparing people of the Mediaeval Ages and modern people in Spain [5]. Sikanjic also made a similar finding in the number of missing teeth in human skeletal remains from the Iron Age in Croatia [6]. Diet and ingredients used in meals (i.e., nutrients) are expected to differ by country. Although it is difficult to generalize, modern people can receive scientific dental care, and tooth extraction can be performed easily and frequently. One cannot say that the dental treatment of tooth extraction was non-existent in the pre-modern times. However, it was likely not performed frequently, and the general public in those times were not as familiar with medical care as the general public of modern time [9].

The average lifespan of Japanese people is estimated to have been less than 15 years in the Jomon period and approximately 20 years in the Edo period [10]. The high mortality rates of infants and young children greatly decreased the average lifespan of the overall population. In these time periods, many adults also lost their lives due to various infections and parasitic diseases. Until the Edo period, Japanese people had a simple and plain diet, except for a small segment of the upper class. Such a diet did not contain much animal protein or fat. Diet in Japanese people began to change due to the introduction of more "American" foods, mainly with the post-war American occupation. Japanese people gradually began to consume more animal protein and fat. It is clearly consistent with the high correlation between increased average lifespan in Japanese people and increased consumption of animal protein and fat (Figures 3 and 4). Japan is currently a country with the longest lifespan in the world. This fact seems to suggest that there is a good balance of the two types of diet, a simple Japanese diet, mainly of vegetables and grains, and a Western-style diet.

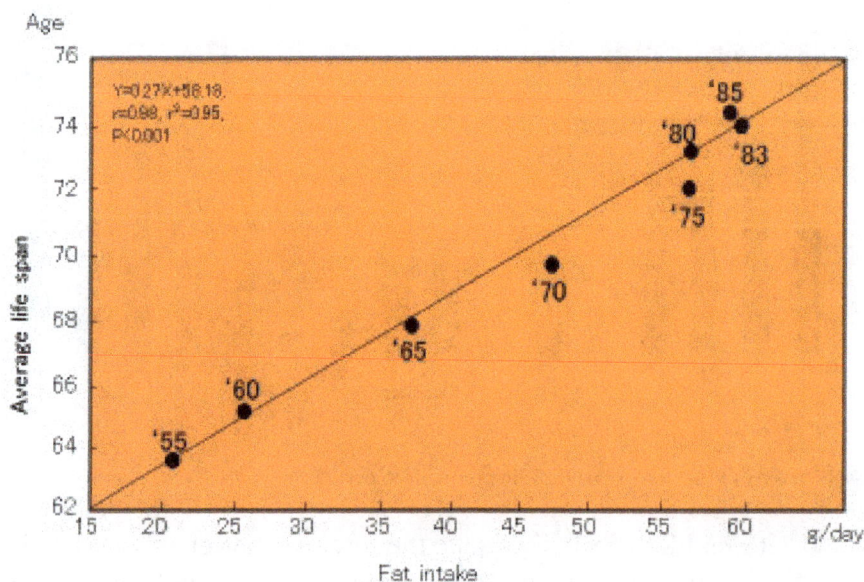

Figure 3. Relation between fat intake and Japanese life span

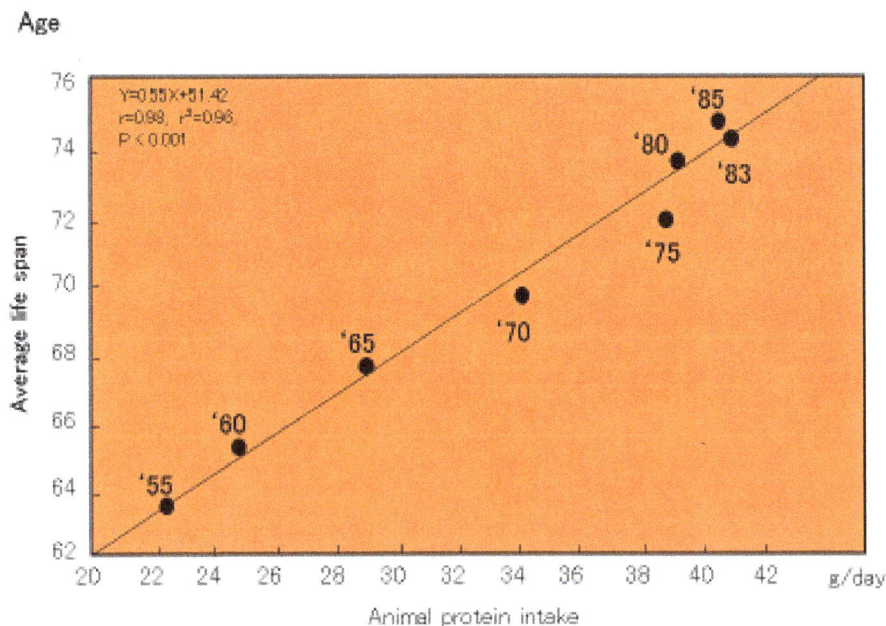

Figure 4. Relation between the animal protein intake and Japanese life span

Intravenous infusion was first introduced to Japan around 1960, and non-parenteral nutrition via gastrostomy was introduced much more recently. There are many restrictions and limitations when using these methods. In the time periods with only pre-modern medical care, the preservation of one's teeth was the only available way for people to get nutrients effectively. Thus, when people lost many of their teeth, they likely faced early death.

2.2. Tooth loss in ancient human skeletal remains from countries other than Japan

How was tooth loss in ancient human skeletal remains from other countries? The status of missing teeth was examined in human skeletal remains of the 3rd-7th centuries from the Yean-ri site in South Korea [11]. There were 2.7 missing teeth in the early middle age individuals and 8 missing teeth in the late middle age individuals, which are not large numbers. The status of missing teeth was also examined in modern Nigerian individuals who lived in the early 20th century and whose skeletal remains are stored at the University of Cambridge [12]. There were 1.3 missing teeth in the early middle age individuals and 3.3 missing teeth in the late middle age individuals, indicating very low numbers. No caries was observed in the examination of a total of 15 Nigerian individuals and 272 teeth. Similarly, when tooth loss was examined in Somali individuals living in the late 19th century to the early 20th century, AMTL was 2.60% in individuals in early middle age [13]. This percentage is a very low value, indicating the loss of at the most 1 tooth out of 32 teeth. In individuals in late middle age, AMTL was 17.02%, which is an approximate loss of 5.4 teeth. Thus, the number of missing teeth clearly increased with aging. There was a significant increase in alveolar bone loss with aging as shown in Table 4, while there was no change in caries rate with aging as shown in Table 5. It is speculated from these results that tooth loss in Somalis was due to periodontal disease and not caries. Although it is difficult to speculate on the details of their diet, they were believed to have had a low intake of simple sugars and carbohydrates. Thus, the diet of Somalis likely consisted of low cariogenic food. The Somali skeletal remains showed that they had periodontal disease from their early middle age. The disease progressed with age and caused alveolar bone loss, eventually leading to bone that could not support the teeth and consequently to tooth loss. The author observed an unexpectedly large number of remaining teeth in the late middle age individuals, much like in the Edo individuals in Japan. It indicated that Somali individuals also had low numbers of missing teeth.

					Tooth type						
	Upper							Lower			
Early middle age	I	C	P	M	Total	I	C	P	M	Total	Grand total
Observed	168	84	170	252	674	130	65	130	195	520	1194
Loss	9	3	1	8	21	0	0	3	7	10	31
SD	0.23	0.19	0.08	0.18	0.17	—	—	0.15	0.19	0.14	0.16
% AMTL	5.36	3.57	0.59	3.17	3.12	0	0	2.31	3.59	1.92	2.60
Early middle age vs Late middle age	$P=0.135$ ns	$P=0.333$ ns	$P<0.01$ L>E	$P<0.001$ L>E	$P<0.001$ L>E	$P<0.001$ L>E	$P<0.05$ L>E	$P=0.051$ ns	$P<0.001$ L>E	$P<0.001$ L>E	$P<0.001$ L>E
Late middle age	I	C	P	M	Total	I	C	P	M	Total	Grand total
Observed	52	26	52	78	208	44	22	43	65	174	382
Loss	7	3	5	18	33	6	3	5	18	32	65
SD	0.32	0.33	0.3	0.42	0.37	0.35	0.35	0.32	0.45	0.39	0.38
% AMTL	13.46	11.54	9.62	23.08	15.87	13.64	13.64	11.63	27.69	18.39	17.02

I: Incisors; C: Canines; P: Premolars; M: Molars in tooth type distribution.

ns: not significant

E: Early middle age; L: Late middle age

Table 5. Antemortem tooth loos (AMTL) of Somali people in Early middle age and Late middle age.

The lifespan remains short in developing countries of the 21st century. Similar types and proportions of disease are thought to have been maintained in modern populations (likely even in present-day populations) as in the populations of 1000-2000 years ago. It is speculated that missing teeth of populations of 1000-2000 years ago were maintained at very low numbers until late middle age despite the presence of periodontal disease, much like ancient human skeletal remains from Japan.

Early middle age				Late middle age				P-value
Tooth type	Observed	Caries	% Caries	Tooth type	Observed	Caries	% Caries	
UI	168	0	0	UI	52	0	0	-
UC	84	0	0	UC	26	0	0	-
UP	170	0	0	UP	52	1	1.92	P=0.537
UM	252	6	2.38	UM	78	0	0	P=0.384
U-total	674	6	0.89	U-total	208	1	0.48	P=0.896
LI	130	0	0	LI	44	0	0	-
LC	65	0	0	LC	22	0	0	-
LP	130	0	0	LP	43	0	0	-
LM	195	4	2.05	LM	65	2	3.08	P=0.991
L-total	520	4	0.77	L-total	174	2	1.15	P=0.994
Grand Total	1194	10	0.84	Grand Total	382	3	0.79	P=0.820

Table 6. Prevalence of dental caries of Somali people in Early middle age and Late middle age.

3. Stress markers and enamel hypoplasia

Stress in modern-day people signifies mainly "psychological stress" in the majority of cases. In ancient skeletal human remains, the focus is on the examination of signs of "physical stress" remaining in bones and teeth as a result of surviving in a very harsh environment. It is desirable to examine the level of such stress not in one or a few individuals but in a group, if possible in at least a few dozen to a few hundred individuals. Otherwise, the stress level in a certain group and differences in stress level among groups cannot be known.

Stress marker might not be a commonly used term. It is a lesion that is used to compare the level of health particularly among groups such as mentioned above. Stress markers on teeth are not very common. Enamel hypoplasia is one such marker and will be discussed below pertaining to ancient human skeletal remains.

Teeth are formed relatively early and enamel matrix is formed at approximately the sixth week of gestation for primary teeth. Enamel matrix formation begins early even for permanent teeth. For example, it begins to form at birth for permanent first molars. Enamel hypoplasia occurs when there is poor enamel formation at such stages. The cause is hypocalcemia due to conditions such as starvation and impaired food intake due to serious disease [14].

Enamel hypoplasia is a useful stress marker because: (1) it is a lesion which is found relatively frequently in ancient human skeletal remains, and (2) it is a lesion that occurs due to environmental factors such as those affecting the nutritional status. Briefly explained, the ancient human skeletal remains that we encounter represent one individual in a few thousands or a few tens of thousands of individuals who lived in the past from a certain time period. They represent a very fortunate discovery and are very important representatives. Therefore, if a disease occurred only in one in a few tens or hundreds of thousands, finding this disease in the excavated remains is greatly affected by chance. Therefore, such disease is not suitable for examining the stress level in a group or comparing the stress level with other groups.

As shown in Figure 5, enamel hypoplasia often appears linearly on the enamel surface. The crowns of healthy teeth should be smooth, but aplasia occurs in depressions of the crowns of teeth with enamel hypoplasia.

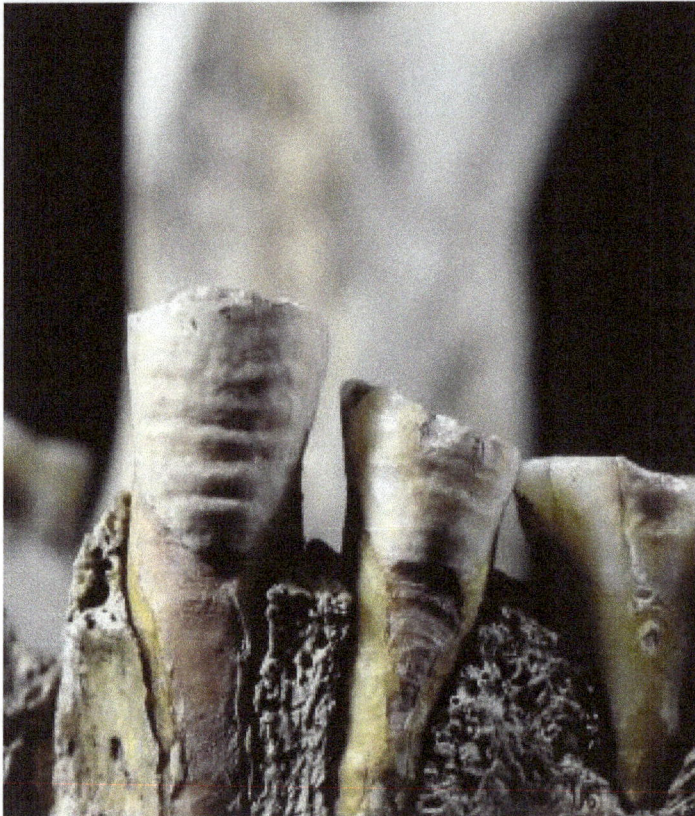

Figure 5. Linear enamel hypoplasia found in Jomon people of Japan

Although there are individual differences, the timing of crown formation by tooth type is roughly the same among individuals. Therefore, when enamel hypoplasia is seen in a certain site of a certain tooth, one can estimate the age at which the enamel hypoplasia occurred. If several lines can be seen in an individual (Figure 5), it can be speculated that this individual experienced multiple bouts of starvation or malnutrition due to serious disease. Some individuals have linear enamel hypoplasia of the entire dentition as in Figure 6. It shows that the individual was exposed to stress causing enamel hypoplasia during crown formation of different tooth types [14]. Therefore, this case is very important as such evidence.

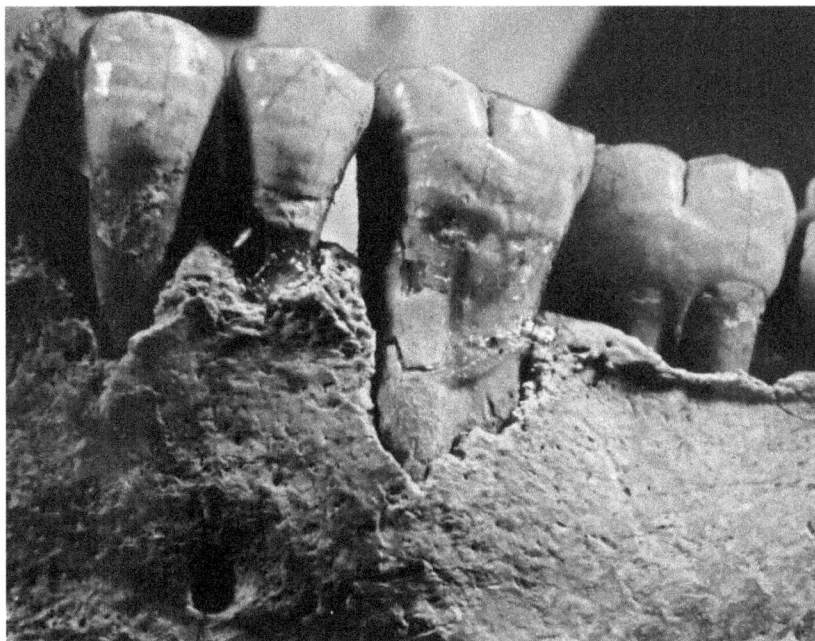

Figure 6. Linear enamel hypoplasia found some tooth type in Jomon people of Japan

When does enamel hypoplasia occur? There have been several studies on this topic, including one by Yamamoto, who examined ancient human skeletal remains of Japanese individuals [15]. According to the study of Yamamoto, enamel hypoplasia occurs repeatedly between 3.5-5.5 years of age in the majority of the cases and very rarely occurs at ages younger than 3 years. Yamamoto gave as reasons for the onset: such stress was likely fatal in individuals at ages younger than 3 years in a pre-modern environment, and even if individuals survived the stress, they could not have tolerated subsequent stress and would have died before the eruption of permanent teeth. In contrast, enamel hypoplasia in modern-day individuals occurs repeatedly at 0-12 months after birth but rarely beyond 34 months [15]. That is, it occurs repeatedly early after birth but rapidly decreases thereafter. Thus, the ancient skeletal remains indicate that timing of hypoplasia differed between ancient people and modern-day people. It is speculated that improved health status, including due to medical advancement, helps modern-day individuals face conditions recorded in crowns as enamel hypoplasia without causing death.

The above findings show that it was very difficult for very young children, particularly infants, to survive in pre-modern times during which bouts of starvation were common and medical care was not advanced. This tendency was likely stronger in more ancient times, and countless young lives must have been lost before these individuals were able to leave any signs of enamel hypoplasia.

Stress markers develop on bones and teeth when individuals continue to survive under a poor environment. If individuals die in a short period of time due to disease or malnutrition, then there will be no stress marker on bones or teeth. For example, when individuals die of acute infections, including dysentery and influenza, it is very difficult to find signs of such infections in excavated bones and teeth. If individuals had chronic diseases such as advanced tuberculosis, leprosy, and syphilis of the bone for a few years to decades, then signs of such diseases will remain in their bones.

The frequency of enamel hypoplasia was 48.1% in the Jomon population, 36.4% in the Kofun population, approximately 60% in the Edo population, and 39.5% in the present-day population of Japan [15]. These numbers seem to indicate that the environment in the Jomon period was better than that in the Edo period. However, these numbers can be explained in another way. When Jomon people suffered various diseases or malnutrition, they likely did not recover and died a short time later. Therefore, they probably did not live long enough to develop enamel hypoplasia, resulting in a lower frequency of enamel hypoplasia in the Jomon period. Edo people also likely lived in a much harsher environment than present-day people. However, medical care and nutritional conditions were improved in the Edo period compared with those in the Jomon period. Therefore, Edo people with various diseases and malnutrition likely had higher chances of survival than Jomon people with such conditions. As a result, signs of enamel hypoplasia remain in individuals from the Edo period. Present-day people can have high-quality medical care and nutrition readily and sufficiently, and the infant mortality rate has consequently decreased. Thus, only a modest frequency of enamel hypoplasia is seen. Therefore, in this type of a situation, one should conclude that a group with a low frequency of stress markers had a worse environment and that a group with a high frequency had a better environment. This phenomenon is called a "paleopathological paradox." One needs to be mindful of this paradox when examining nutritional conditions, health status, and the difference in frequency of disease among groups or time periods.

What are the frequencies of enamel hypoplasia in various countries? When the frequency of enamel hypoplasia was examined in former inhabitants of what is now the State of Illinois in the U.S., it was 45% in the excavated individuals from the hunting and gathering period, 60% in the excavated individuals from the transition to the agricultural period, and a high frequency of 80% in the excavated individuals from the agricultural period [16]. Similarly, when the frequency was examined in former inhabitants of what is now Ohio, it was higher in the excavated individuals from the agricultural period than those from the hunting and gathering period [17, 18]. These findings indicate that poor harvests more greatly affected people in an agricultural society than frequent food shortages affected people in a hunting and gathering society. In addition, the agricultural people who lived in these areas had a diet which depended heavily on corn. Such a diet resulted in increased caloric intake and nutritional quantity but decreased animal protein intake and nutritional quality. Weaning diets were deficient in protein, and nutritional stress occurred such as diarrhea due to bacterial infection. Some researchers interpret the high frequency of enamel hypoplasia as a result of increased population density in the agricultural period, leading to a higher risk for infection and increased environmental stress such as outbreaks of endemic diseases [19, 20].

The author of this paper is not in agreement with the above explanations. There is no evidence that a hunter-gatherer economy enabled people to maintain necessary and sufficient proteins. There is also no evidence that people in an agricultural economy had repeated poor harvests and had lower animal protein intake than people in a hunter-gatherer economy. The term "hunters and gatherers" gives the image of hunting. However, it is speculated that people in a hunter-gatherer economy did not necessary have sufficient animal-derived foods, and the majority of their diet consisted of plant-derived foods. Even natural-born hunters like lions have very low hunting success rates. Therefore, it is valid opinion that hunters and gatherers must have had great difficulties maintaining a constant intake of animal protein even with human intelligence and use of tools. The diet of an agricultural economy could not have consisted entirely of plant-derived foods. Instead, it is speculated that hunting must have continued, and its techniques must have evolved from previous time periods to the agricultural period. Therefore, people must have continued to consume animal-derived foods in the agricultural period.

Even when societies transitioned from a hunting-gathering type to an agricultural type, it is very unlikely that the consumption of animal protein decreased sharply. Instead, the afore-mentioned enamel hypoplasia frequencies should be interpreted in the following ways: the types of people who were unable to survive in a hunter-gatherer society were more likely to survive in an agricultural society, and the average lifespan, an index of cumulative stress, increased.

4. TMD in human skeletal remains from the Edo period in Japan

Prolonged retention of primary teeth rarely poses clinical problems in modern people if these teeth are extracted and the eruptive paths of permanent teeth are normalized. A report in a Japanese journal has shown that when primary teeth were retained beyond the normal period, their extraction resulted in gradual improvement of TMD and in normal occlusion. In the field of physical anthropology, very few report has been published that simultaneously discussed prolonged retention of primary teeth, temporomandibular joint (TMJ) arthritis, and TMD [21]. The material discussed in this section was skeletal human remains from the Edo period (17-19th centuries) in Japan. The mandible showed signs of TMJ arthritis and TMD likely due to bilateral primary second molars. The skeletal remains were excavated from the Suhgen temple site in Shinjuku-ku in Tokyo and were of a woman in the early part of early middle age. Retention of primary molars was observed in the left and right mandible (Figure 7). Since first premolars were present anterior to them, the over-retained primary teeth were both believed to be primary second molars. Radiographs showed no formation of left or right second premolars, confirming that they were missing congenitally (Figures 8a and 8b). It was speculated that bilateral primary second molars remained in adulthood because second premolars were missing congenitally. Other permanent mandibular teeth, including the third molars, were erupted bilaterally, and it is consistent with the individual being in the early part of early middle age. Bilateral primary molars had more severe occlusal attrition of the distal area than on the mesial area, and dentin was markedly exposed. The occlusal attrition of the mesial area was confined to near the proximal aspect adjacent to the first premolar.

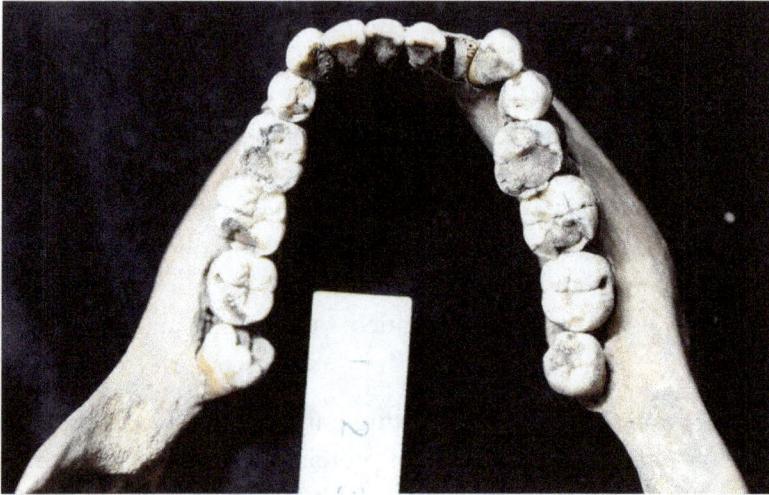

Figure 7. Persistence of both sides of second deciduous molars.

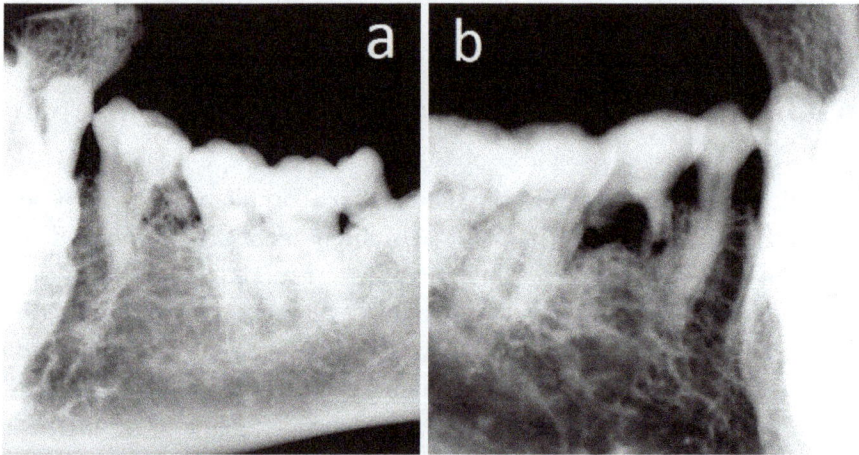

Figure 8. The lack of permanent second premolars are admitted in the roentgenograms. a: right side, b: left side, respectively. a: right mandibular condyle is normal. b: left mandibular condyle has caused the deformity by TMJ arthritis.

The right mandibular condyle was normal, but TMJ arthritis had developed in the left mandibular condyle with overall deformation (Figures 9a and 9b). It was of minimum expression under the Rando and Waldron classification [22]. The right mandibular fossa was normal. In the left mandibular fossa, a new articular facet had formed accompanying inflammation and deformation of the mandibular condyle, and it was evident that TMJ arthritis and accompanying TMD had developed (Figures 10a and 10b).

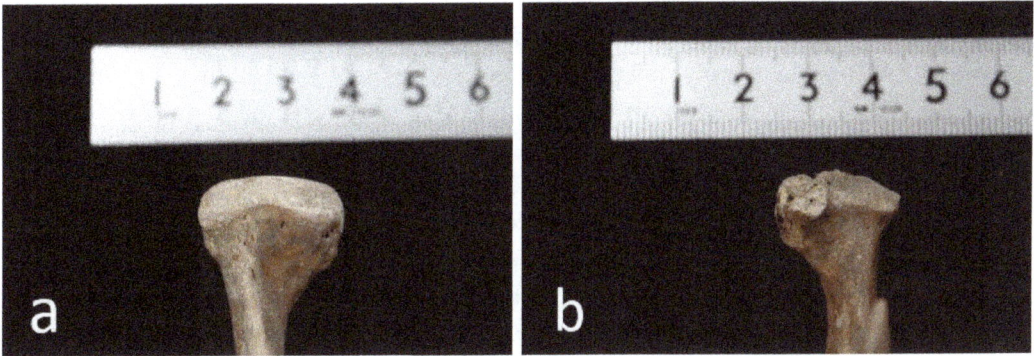

Figure 9. a: mandibular fossa of both sides. b: left mandibular fossa forms the false joint (arrow) and porosity is recognized in frame area.

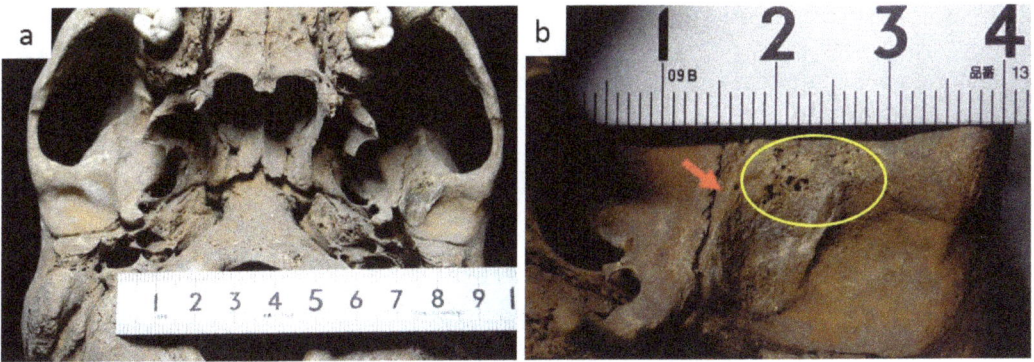

Figure 10. Periostitis found in the alveolar bone at right second deciduous molar (a) and left second deciduous molar (b).

There was bilateral periostitis of the alveolar bone supporting the primary teeth (Figures 11a and 11b). Periostitis was severe in the areas with over-retained primary second molars, and there was mild periostitis in all other areas, which was almost the entire maxilla and mandible.

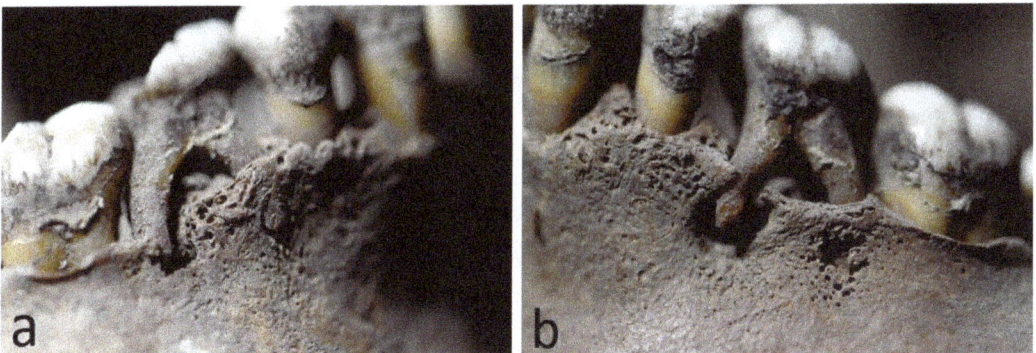

Figure 11. Slight periostitis is admitted in the widespread area of the alveolar bone.

Sumiya reported that the prevalence of prolonged retention was 0.58% for primary second molars in both Japanese men and women aged 21-25 years [23]. Onizuka examined 151 teeth in 106 individuals with over-retained primary teeth who were aged 14-47 years and reported that 63% had one over-retained tooth and 32% had two over-retained teeth [24]. It should be noted that over-retained teeth occurred symmetrically in the left and right sides of the maxilla or mandible in 33 of 34 patients with two over-retained teeth, indicating a very high proportion of patients [24]. The most commonly over-retained tooth was the primary second molar at 52.3% [24]. In the individual from the Suhgen temple site, there was prolonged retention of two mandibular primary second molars with bilaterally symmetry. The occurrence rate was 0.19% based on simple calculation, suggesting that such prolonged retention occurred in approximately 2 in 1000 adults. When one takes into account that the excavated skeletal remains were of the Edo period, this individual can be said to represent a valuable case of over-retained primary teeth in ancient human skeletal remains.

Although some reports have discussed that over-retained primary teeth can frequently cause TMD, treatment such as extraction of such teeth has been reported to improve the symptoms. In the individual from the Suhgen temple site, occlusal attrition was observed in the distal area of the left and right first molars. In the right first molar, the occlusal surface gently sloped upward from the distal to the mesial direction until there was no attrition. One area of the left first molar showed severe attrition where its distal area contacted the left second molar. It is nearly impossible to reproduce an accurate antemortem occlusion using a mandible and maxilla without soft tissue. However, there was likely abnormal occlusal force on the areas with attrition. When the maxillary dentition was examined, the teeth had normal positions in the left and right molar regions and there was slight attrition confined to the enamel. Attrition was confined to the lingual aspect for the left and right maxillary first molars. In this individual, the findings were strongly suggestive of malocclusion such as cusp-to-cusp occlusion. It is not known whether TMD occurred at a transition period from primary teeth to permanent teeth or after eruption of all permanent teeth. In any case, prolonged retention of primary second molars was thought to have somehow contributed to the development of TMD.

There are limitations in discussing TMD based on archeological materials, but there can be reports of new valuable cases of archeological materials. Modern-day individuals can have prolonged retention of primary teeth causing TMD and can have concurrent periodontal disease. Therefore, it is desirable to appropriately treat individuals with such conditions in modern clinical dental medicine. The material from the Suhgen temple site was an excavated archeological sample, but the implication of its findings can be important in modern dental medicine.

5. Conclusions

This paper discussed three topics from the perspective of physical anthropology which handles ancient human skeletal remains: antemortem tooth loss and problems of periodontal disease and caries, enamel hypoplasia as a stress marker, and occurrence of TMD due to prolonged retention of primary teeth. There are many other oral diseases in ancient skeletal remains that the author of this paper would like to discuss but was unable to, due to limitation of space. The diseases discussed in this paper are all in the oral region and have afflicted people from a few thousand years ago until the present day, i.e., diseases which have also afflicted our ancestors. The author hopes that the readers were able to appreciate that many new findings can be obtained from examination of diseases in the past. It is important to focus on the present to save patients who suffer from modern-day diseases. However, when one examines only the present, one will likely be unable to properly envision dental health of the future. The author is of the opinion that "knowing the past" or "learning from the past" is a very important point. Modern humans have existed for a long time, the ancestors of whom emerged about 7 million years ago. Thus, humans have a long past and modern humans should be thought of as being on the leading edge of this long human history.

Cooperation of physical anthropologists will be important in the creation of guidelines in modern medicine and future oral health. Such an effort can organically link the past, present, and future for the first time and can contribute to a better future. Another hope of this author is that the information and findings of this paper will be useful to many readers.

Author details

Hisashi Fujita*

Address all correspondence to: rxh05535@nifty.com

Department of Bioanthropology, Niigata College of Nursing, Japan

References

[1] Sakai S. Japanese History from the diseases. Tokyo: Kodansha; 2014. (in Japanese)

[2] Trinkaus E.; Pathology and Posture of the La Chapelle-aux-Saints Neandertal. Am. J. Phys. Anthropol. 1985, 67, 19-41.

[3] Trinkaus E. The Shanidar Neandertals. Academic Press, New York, USA, 1983.

[4] Nelson GC, Lukacs JR, Yule P. Dates, Caries, and Early Tooth Loss During the Iron Age of Oman. Am J. Phys. Anthropol. 1999, 108, 333-343.

[5] Lopez B, Pardinas AF, Gacia-Vazquez E. Dopico E. Socio-cultural fractures in dental diseases in the Medieval and early Modern Age of northern Spain. Homo. 2012, 63, 21-42.

[6] Sikanjic PR. Bioarchaeology research in Croatia—a historical review. Coll Anthropol. 2005, 29(2): 763-768.

[7]   Fujita H. The number of missing teeth in people of the Edo period in Japan in the 17th to 19th centuries. Gerodontol. 2012, 29, e520-e524.

[8]   Oyamada J, Igawa K, Manabe Y, Kato K, Matsushita T, Rokutanda A, Kitagawa Y. Preliminary analysis of regional differences in dental pathology of early modern commoners in Japan. Anthropol. Sci. 2010, 118, 1-8.

[9]   Takehara T, Sakashita R, Fujita H, Matsushita T, Simoyama A. History of dental caries. : Tokyo; Sunashobo, 2001. (in Japanese)

[10] Fujita H. Were the Jomon People healthy or not? Speculation of total health condition of ancient people. J. Lipid Nutrition, 2007 16(2), 205-210.

[11] Fujita H., Suzuki, T., Shoda, S., Kawakubo, Y., Ohno, K., Giannakopoulou, P. and Harihara, S.: Contribution on antemortem tooth loss (AMTL) and dental attrition to oral palaeopathology in the human skeletal series from the Yean-ri site, South Korea. International Journal of Archaeology, 2013 1:1-5.

[12] Fujita H. Dental Diseases and Stress Markers on Crania in the Early Modern People of Nigeria. Japanese Journal of Gerodontology, 2013 28(1): 10-19.

[13] Fujita H. Health status in early modern Somali people from their skeletal remains. Int J Archaeol 2014, 2(3), 1-5.

[14] Jalevik B, Noren JG. Enamel hypomineralization of permanent first molars: a morphological study and survey of possible aetiological factors. Int. J. Paediatr. Dent., 2000 10: 278-289.

[15] Yamamoto M. Enamel Hypoplasia of the Permanent Teeth in Japanese from the Jomon to the Modern Periods. J. Anthrop. Soc. Nippon 1988 96(4) 417-433.

[16] Goodman AH, Armelagos GJ, Rose JC. Enamel hypoplasia as as indicators of stress in three prehistoric populations from Illinois. Human Biol. 1980 52: 515-528.

[17] Sciulli PW, Developmental abnormalities of the permanent dentition in prehistoric Ohio Valley Amerindians. Am. J. Phys. Anthropol., 1978 48: 193-198.

[18] Cook DC. Subsistence and health in the Lower Illinois Valley: Osteological evidence. In: Cohen M and Aemelagos GJ (ed.) Paleopathology at the Origins of Agriculture. Academic Press, 1984 235-269.

[19] Lallo JW, Rose JC. Patterns of stress, diseases and mortality in two prehistoric populations from North America. J. Human Evolution, 1979 8: 323-335.

[20] Cassidy CM. Nutrition and health in agriculturalist and hunter-gatherers. In: Jerome NW, Kandel RF, Pelto GH (ed.) Nutritional Anthropology, Redgrave Press, 1980 117-145.

[21] Fujita H, Suzuki T, Harihara S. Simultaneous Dental Anomalies (Polyanomalodontia) in Mediaeval Japanese Skeletal Remains. Jpn. J. Oral. Biol. 1997 39: 257-262.

[22] Rando C, Waldron T. TMJ Osteoarthritis: A New Approach to Diagnosis. Am. J. Phys. Anthropol. 2012 148: 45-53

[23] Sumiya Y. Statistic Study on Dental Anomalies in the Japanese. J. Anthropol. Soc. Nippon. 1959 64: 215-233. (in Japanese)

[24] Onizuka Y. Statistical Observation on the Multiple Cases (106 Cases) of the Retained Deciduous Teeth. Kyushu Shika Gakkai Zasshi 1979 33: 52-67. (in Japanese)

5

Oral Health Care Needs in the Geriatric Population

Derek S J D'Souza

1. Introduction

During the first decade of the 21st century, medical advances have increased life expectancy significantly, especially in the developed world. Life-threatening infectious diseases have notably reduced and many chronic diseases can be better controlled by long-term medications and surgery. Improvement in the understanding and treatment of oral health issues has also resulted in the definite improvement in oral health. There were 390 million people in USA aged over 65 years as per the figures of the 1998 World Health Report and this figure is estimated to double by 2025. In many developing countries, particularly in South America and Asia, it is predicted that there will be an increase of up to 300% of the elderly population in the next decade. By 2050, there will be 2 billion people over the age of 60, with almost 80% living in developing countries [1]. The growth in this group of citizens is staggering, posing tremendous challenges to those involved in planning the care that is necessary for this ageing population. At the end of 1950s, the population over seventy years of age was mainly edentulous. However with better access to oral health care and better understanding of oral diseases and newer treatment modalities, the mean number of retained teeth had increased to 14 by 2010 and this can be expected to rise further in the years to come. This new group of partially dentate elderly who carry the burden of chronic disease and are on multiple medications, presents a new set of problem areas to the clinician. However, in the some of the lesser developed countries the situation and the problems are different. Though life expectancy has increased the oral health status has not kept pace. Thus there is significant loss of teeth in the elderly and this reduced dentition also affects food intake leading to vitamin deficiency or even malnutrition. There is an urgent need to understand the oral health care needs of these different groups of geriatric patients as well as improve the quality of prosthetic rehabilitation.

2. Age changes in the elderly

Among the aged there is a high prevalence of co-morbidities and numerous barriers to care. Oral health conditions include: High caries prevalence; Advanced Periodontal disease/ loss of attachment and poor oral hygiene; Edentulousness and limited masticatory functioning; Denture related conditions, ill fitting removable dentures; Head and neck cancer or co-morbidities due to radiation or chemotherapy; Xerostomia; Craniofacial pain and discomfort [1, 2].

The oral mucosa becomes thinner and more vulnerable to external injuries with advancing age. Thus the prevalence of soft tissue changes has been reported to be high among the elderly. Ill-fitting dentures are also known to increase the risk of oral mucosal changes. There is a well established association between prosthetic factors, denture hygiene and presence of oral mucosal lesions in the elderly.

Intake of multiple medications results in decreased salivary flow, as a side effect, which further compromises the health of the fragile oral mucosa. Saliva neutralizes the production of acids by oral microflora and also helps in tooth remineralisation. Saliva has numerous protective benefits for the teeth and the oral mucosa due to its content of immunoglobulin A and lactoferrin [3]. Reduction in salivary flow results in an increased number of oral micro-flora as well as their metabolic by-products in the oral cavity. This leads to an increase in the caries index and also results in increased tooth loss to periodontal diseases. Changes in physical and mental status also manifest as a deterioration of co-ordination and motor skills that are necessary for maintenance of proper oral hygiene. These reduced oral hygiene practices further contributes to prolific growth of harmful oral microflora [4, 5].

Changes in diet as well as altered taste and smell all play their part in reducing the amount of food intake of most of the elderly. When economic factors or the standardized diets provided in hospices or other institutions for the elderly are taken into consideration it becomes obvious of how difficult it is to meet the nutritional goals in the elderly. There is also higher catabolic rates and increase in demand for certain vital nutrients to keep pace with the overall age changes in the body. Thus it is paramount that a close check be kept on the overall nutritional status as well as the appearance of signs and symptoms of malnutrition [6].

3. Residual Ridge Resorption (RRR)

Residual ridge resorption (RRR) is a term that is used to describe the changes which affect the alveolar ridge following tooth extractions, and which continue even long after healing of the extraction socket. The most significant feature of this healing process is that the residual bony architecture of the maxilla and mandible undergoes a life-long catabolic remodelling. The rate of reduction in size of the residual ridge is maximum in the first three months and then gradually tapers off. However, bone resorption activity continues throughout life at a slower rate, resulting in loss of varying amount of jaw structure, ultimately leaving the patient a 'dental cripple' [7].

The speed and direction of alveolar bone loss is not similar in maxilla and mandible. The changes seen in the mandible are quicker and more dramatic changes due to the unique tear-drop cross-sectional shape of the mandible. In mandible resorption proceeds more in labio-lingual and vertical directions. The net result is that the mandible appear to move downward and outward. In the maxilla the changes occur evenly around the dental arch, but more on buccal and labial side than on the palatal side. This results in the maxilla appearing to move inward and upwards. This differing age changes in the two arches is the reason that there is a relative prognathism of the edentulous mandible seen after many years of edentulousness. Unlike in maxilla, the speed of bone loss in mandible is different in different parts of the jaw i.e. distal parts of the residual ridge resorb faster than the anterior region [8].

Multiple factors can affect RRR. Age and gender differences are well documented; there is a clear correlation between mandibular RRR and females. Systemic factors like osteoporosis, diseases related to thyroid function, medication, general lifestyle and local oral and prosthetic factors might all influence RRR. Due to resorption the mental foramen and alveolar nerve can finally relocate on the crest of the alveolar bone. As a result of this, denture's functional properties can seriously deteriorate and wearing a mandibular denture can be a very painful experience. Functional stability, a combination of stability and retention of the denture, is strongly affected by the degree of RRR and condition of the denture, especially in the lower jaw. As a consequence of RRR, location of mandibular related muscle attachments are situated closer to the crest of mandibular bone [9]. In combination with age-related muscle atrophy and dry mouth, this may lead to a situation where denture-wearing experience, especially of worn-out dentures, is very unsatisfying and frustrating.

4. Prosthetic rehabilitation in the elderly

Poor retention and stability of complete dentures is one of the main dental related complaints in edentulous persons. Poor retention is often related to loss of alveolar bone support. Reasons for residual ridge resorption (RRR) are multiple and may vary among individuals. It begins after extraction of teeth and progresses at varying speed for the rest of the life. Both local and systemic factors may affect the rate of RRR.

Total or partial loss of natural teeth as such does not necessarily mean that the missing teeth have to be replaced with dental prostheses. The elderly often consider it acceptable to have a few missing teeth as long as they are can be socially and functionally satisfactory. Thus they delay in reporting for dental treatment and this further complicates their chances for complete rehabilitation. The clinician's objective plan for rehabilitation alone is not considered justified enough to undergo treatment. Missing anterior teeth are often sought to be replaced immediately for esthetic reasons but there are no generally accepted criteria for replacing missing teeth, especially in the posterior region. The maximum masticatory efficiency has been seen to be in the region of the premolars and first molar and the patients adapt accordingly if other teeth are lost. Current consensus appears to be that a minimum of four functional occlusal units in shortened dental arches are sufficient to maintain the healthy natural function of the dentition. Patients find it easier to adapt by changing their intake to softer foods or elimination of foods from their diet that are difficult to masticate. This leads to a state of gradual and progressive tooth loss till the patient becomes totally edentulous and then perforce has to opt for the "complete dentures" which are often seen as a dismal symbol that the person is 'aged'.

Complete upper and lower dentures have been the most common form of prosthetic rehabilitation in the totally edentulous group of aged persons. Conventional complete dentures are still the most acceptable and economically affordable form of prosthetic rehabilitation especially in developing countries. Extreme old age, long travel time or inability to travel to the nearest dental clinic and low income are the primary reasons for inadequate prosthetic treatment of edentulous persons [10].

Implant-supported dentures based on osseointegrated titanium implants are the gold standard in dental rehabilitation. Patients who are economically 'well-off' have the option of choosing implant supported over-dentures. These are significantly more acceptable and masticatory function can be restored to a great extent. A well designed mandibular over-denture supported by osseointegrated implants, will enhance the whole masticatory experience more significantly by increasing biting force and improving the biting and chewing function [11]. Today, implant procedures are well-documented to replace missing teeth or to provide retention for complete dentures. Adequate number of implants if placed early can even slow down the inevitable RRR. From the medical point of view there is limited contraindication for the use of osseointegrated implants, but the majority of implant treatment still remain beyond the reach of the majority of elderly.

There has been a noteworthy change in oral health care planning, in that the earlier concept of replacement of every missing tooth is no longer is considered as essential. In subjects with reduced natural dentition, as long as there is sufficient masticatory efficiency to meet the nutritional requirements of the individual and the aesthetic concerns have been fulfilled, there is no need to replace all the missing teeth. Thus, a shortened dental arch (SDA) as such does not dictate an urgent need for prosthetic treatment. As long as there is occlusal stability and functional occlusion is maintained, free-end removable partial dentures (RPD) may not provide significant masticatory advantages and may be avoided.

Rehabilitation using RPD's demands a high level of competence on the part of the clinician and a regular follow-up from the patient. These dentures can actually cause more harm than good if long term oral health is not maintained and the resultant forces generated by these prostheses can be highly detrimental to the health of the remaining teeth. Those patients who have been provided with RPD's need regular follow-up and care to ensure that their dentures are functioning as planned and necessary oral care is being maintained. Failure to properly maintain the RPD's in some cases may increase the risk of caries and periodontal disease for the remaining dentition thus worsening oral health [12]. It is important to keep in mind that RPD patients need regular surveillance through a recall system. This is not an easy task when dealing with elderly patients, bearing in mind that they form the component of population that faces the greatest number of barriers to oral health services.

Today, the ever-increasing number of geriatric cases requiring oral rehabilitation necessitates new treatment strategies. There may be a difference of opinion between the treating clinician and the patients regarding the treatment plan and objectives and this may complicate treatment planning. In most cases, patients desire good aesthetics and comfort, whereas the dental surgeon would often stress on the importance of good functionality. The minimum number of teeth needed to satisfy functional and social demands varies individually. This depends on multiple local and systemic factors, such as periodontal condition of the remaining teeth, occlusal forces and a person's adaptive capacity and age. Thus, the greatest challenge for the clinician is to choose between either treating the patient with the risk of producing iatrogenic disease, or, not treating the patient and resulting in reduced nutritional intake or gastrointestinal disorders. Economic factors also play a significant role in the choice of treatment as the material costs are normally prohibitively high. Even health insurance schemes provide limited cover as far as oral rehabilitation schemes are concerned. This further widens the gap between ideal and essential treatment and it is the geriatric patient who ends up facing the worst outcome in such a scenario.

5. Denture hygiene and oral lesions

Numerous mucosal lesions such as denture stomatitis, angular cheilitis, flabby ridge, irritation hyperplasia, traumatic ulcers and even cancer have been associated with the prolonged use of unhygenic or grossly worn-out removable dentures. Up to seventy-six per cent of all oral mucosal lesions have reported to be inflammatory or reactive in nature [13].

Candida albicans is the most common microorganism related to denture wearing. Several studies have been conducted to explore the relationship between yeasts and denture-induced stomatitis. Close correlation between the use of dentures at night and smoking has also been reported. The influence of patient's age, denture hygiene, use of drugs and denture wearing habits has been well documented. Also a low salivary flow rate may predispose the oral mucosa to the pathological changes because of its association with the presence of yeasts inside the mouth cavity. The number and type of several oral microflora have also been shown to be elevated in denture wearers and in the elderly suffering from xerostomia [14].

Against this background the role of plaque removal cannot be stressed enough. Older people seem to be generally well informed of the importance of good oral and dental hygiene and their effect on oral health, but less aware of the poor results of their well-meaning cleaning efforts. Most older citizens brush their denture under running water at least once a day, but with the age-related reduced manual dexterity the outcome is hardly ever good. It is obvious that written and verbal information alone is not enough to establish positive oral hygiene behaviour and results. Indeed, repetitive cleaning demonstrations and motivation sessions may be the only way to attain longer lasting changes.

Trauma induced by ill-fitting dentures has been supposed to be the main reason for "denture sore mouth", and tissue hyperplasia. Even with new dentures, ulcers may develop very fast often within few days after fitting of the denture [15, 16]. Thus, denture-associated ulcers are relatively common and patients should be advised to report regularly for follow-up every four to six weeks for new dentures and every six months thereafter. This will ensure that there is immediate intervention to prevent any trauma from age changes of the oral mucosa under the dentures.

In the end there seems to be many conflicting opinions on the nature of oral mucosal lesions. The principles concerning the criteria for treatment needs and preventive treatment methods have been, however, agreed by the majority of authors. Some oral mucosal lesions may be avoided by regular examinations and adjustments of dentures, good oral and denture hygiene and wearing the dentures only during the day [11].

6. Oral health care planning for the geriatric population

Ageing is inevitable, irreversible and a reality that all have to deal with. As people get older, oral health planning needs to refocus its objectives so that they are sustainable with regard to the general health and financial circumstances of the elderly. It is important that people need to have access to oral health care that is based on preventive concepts and be actively involved in making choices about their oral health right from the fifth and sixth decade of life. This will ensure that they can attain a level of oral health that can be maintained into older age [17, 18].

To make this a reality it is essential to utilize the full spectrum of oral health care workers (dental surgeons and specialists, dental hygienists, dental technicians and dental auxiliary staff) in health care set-ups for the elderly [19].

To ensure sustainable change in any oral health scenario, it is vital that consumers and communities be actively involved in decision making about oral health, and empowered to maintain their oral and general health and wellbeing. Current information on the incidence, distribution and determinants of oral diseases must be used for evidence-based planning on the effectiveness and cost effectiveness of oral health intervention. For this national and local oral health surveys must be carried out as they can provide the latest and authentic data about all aspects of oral health status, disease, and their determinants [20, 21].

People with cognitive impairment face a higher risk of oral diseases. Any impairment in maintenance of adequate oral hygiene will result in high caries index and poor periodontal conditions. This increases the cost and complexity of providing oral health services in community, hospice and old-age homes. Co-morbid general health conditions also complicate the effective delivery of medical care services. Reduced masticatory efficiency affects nutrition and can cause reduction in body weight. All these must be factored in while planning, execution and maintenance of any health plan for the eldely

As age advances, there is a gradual decrease in immunity which along with physiological changes and multiple risk factors manifests as an increased risk of infectious disease. Infections such as pneumococcal, influenza, tetanus, and zoster are more common among the older generation. These infections are major causes of morbidity and mortality and are responsible for a large number of deaths and hospitalizations among the elderly. Communicable diseases like influenza and pneumonia are the fifth leading cause of death among elderly persons. Among the many infections to which the elderly are prone, some can be prevented by administration of suitable vaccines. Vaccination of the elderly can be one of the most effective and economic methods means of prevention of long term disease, disability, or death resulting from communicable illnesses [22].

There is an urgent need to train the entire oral health team to meet the needs (including oral health promotion) of older people [19]. A multidisciplinary team approach is needed, involving a complete team of oral health specialists & other primary health care providers (medical and allied health). The poor oral health status of people in residential aged care hospices is clear evidence that the requisite objectives are not achieved with current health planning. There is a need for a fresh approach to ensure that appropriate medical and oral health treatment needs are met within residential facilities for geriatric individuals [23 – 25].

7. Conclusion

Oral health while being important at all stages of life assumes greater value at extreme old age. Worldwide, people are living longer lives as a result of better understanding of disease processes, health concerns, and improvements in overall standards of hygiene and living conditions. Paradoxically, this does not signify that they are necessarily living healthier lives-chronic systemic diseases including oral diseases are on the rise. A decline in oral health is manifested as higher numbers of missing teeth, rise in caries index, and an increase in the prevalence rates of periodontal disease, xerostomia and oral pre-cancer/cancer. Non-communicable diseases are fast becoming the leading causes of disability and mortality, and in the near future health and social policy-makers will face tremendous challenges posed by the rapidly increasing burden of chronic diseases in old age.

The negative impact of poor oral conditions on the quality of life of older adults is an important public health issue, that must be addressed by health care planners at all levels. The need of the hour is to translate knowledge into action programmes for the oral health of older people. It is the responsibility of National health planners to develop policies and set priorities and targets for satisfactory oral health. National public health programmes should incorporate oral health promotion and disease prevention based on the common risk factors approach. In developing countries the challenges to provision of effective oral health care are predominantly high because of a variety of factors related to vast populations and the resultant disparity between the rich and the poor. In developed countries too, oral health services need to be revised to take a preventive approach when considering the oral care needs of older people. Funding for better research for optimum oral health should focus beyond just the biomedical and clinical aspects of oral disease. Private-Public partnerships must be encouraged to allow research and efforts to translate science into practice. Education and continuous training must ensure that oral health care providers have the requisite skills and a thorough understanding of the biomedical and psychosocial aspects of care for geriatric group of patients. It is imperative for all of us to undertake whatever we can do to ensure that the oral health care needs of the aged are met before it is too late. A sustainable plan to mitigate the spread of oral disease and illness in older adults should be strengthened by means of an organized, affordable, comprehensive oral health service which can be easily accessed by all.

Author details

Derek S J D'Souza[*]

Address all correspondence to: dsjdsouza@gmail.com

Pune, India

References

[1] Improving oral health amongst the elderly. World Health Organization Geneva. http://www.who.int/oral_health/action/groups/en/index1.html

[2] Shah N. Oral health care system for elderly in India. Geriatrics and Gerontology International 2004; 4: S162– S164.

[3] Bagg J. The oral micro flora and dental plaque. Essentials of microbiology for dental students. Oxford: Oxford University Press: 1999; 229 – 310

[4] Bhaskar SN. Oral pathology in the dental office: study of 20,575 biopsy specimens. JADA 1968; 76:761-71.

[5] Avlund K, Holm-Pedersen P, Schroll M. Functional ability and oral health among older people: A longitudinal study from age 75 to 80. J Am Geriatr Soc 2001; 49:954-62

[6] Marshall TA, Warren JJ, Hand JS, Xie X-J, Stumbo PJ. Oral health, nutrient intake and dietary quality in the very old. J Am Dent Assoc 2002; 133:1369-79.

[7] Atwood DA. Reduction of residual ridge: a major oral disease entity. J Prosthet Dent 1971; 26(3):266-79.

[8] Tallgren A. The continuing reduction of alveolar residual ridges in complete denture wearers: A mixed-longitudinal study covering 25 years. J Prosth Dent 1972; 27:120-32

[9] Nishimura I, Atwood DA. Knife-edge residual ridge: a clinical report. J Prosthet Dent 1994 Mar; 71(3):231-4.

[10] Bernier S, Shotwell J, Razzoog M. Clinical evaluation of complete dentures therapy: Examiner consistency. J Prosthet Dent 1984; 51(5):703-08.

[11] Langer A, Michman J, Seifert I. Factors influencing satisfaction with complete dentures in geriatric patients. J Prosthet Dent 1961; 11:1019-31.

[12] Vermeulen AH, Keltjens HM, Van't Hof MA, Kayser AF. Ten-year evaluation of removable partial dentures: survival rates based on retreatment, not wearing and replacement. J Prosthet Dent 1996 Sep; 76(3):267-72.

[13] Ritchie GM. A report of dental findings in a survey of geriatric patients. Journal of Dentistry 1973; 1:106-12.

[14] Budtz-Jörgensen E. Clinical aspects of Candida infection in denture wearers. J Am Dent Assoc 1978; 42: 619-23.

[15] Ettinger RL. The aetiology of inflammatory papillary hyperplasia. J Prosthet Dent 1975; 34:254-61.

[16] Bastiaan RJ. Denture sore mouth. Aetiological aspects and treatment. Aust Dent J 1976; 21:375-82.

[17] Chalmers JM. Oral diseases in older adults. In: Chalmers JM et al. Ageing and Dental Health. AIHW Dental Statistics and Research Series No. 19. Adelaide: The University of Adelaide. 1999.

[18] Chalmers JM. Oral health promotion for our ageing Australian population. Australian Dental Journal 2003; 48(1): 2-9.

[19] Hopcraft MS, Morgan MV, Satur JG, Wright FA. Utilizing dental hygienists to undertake dental examination and referral in residential aged care facilities. Community Dent Oral Epidemiol. 2011 Aug; 39(4):378-84.

[20] Adachi M, Ishihara K, Abe S, Okuda K, Ishikawa T. Effect of professional oral health care on the elderly living in nursing homes. Oral Surg Oral Med Oral Pathol Oral Radiol Endod. 2002 Aug; 94(2):191-5.

[21] Kokubu K, Senpuku H, Tada A, Saotome Y, Uematsu H. Impact of routine oral care on opportunistic pathogens in the institutionalized elderly. J Med Dent Sci. 2008 Mar; 55(1):7-13.

[22] Verma R, Khanna P, Chawla S. Vaccines for the elderly need to be introduced into the immunization program in India. Hum Vaccin Immunother. 2014 Jun 23; 10(8). [Epub ahead of print]

[23] Morino T, Ookawa K, Haruta N, Hagiwara Y, Seki M. Effects of professional oral health care on elderly: randomized trial. Int J Dent Hyg. 2014 Nov; 12(4): 291- 7.

[24] Ishikawa A, Yoneyama T, Hirota K, Miyake Y, Miyatake K. Professional oral health care reduces the number of oropharyngeal bacteria. J Dent Res. 2008 Jun; 87(6):594-8.

[25] Petersen PE, Kandelman D, Arpin S and Ogawa H. Global oral health of older people
      – Call for public health action. Community Dental Health (2010) 27, (Supplement 2)
      257–268.

6

Infant Oral Health

Preetika Chandna and Vivek K. Adlakha

1. Introduction

Infancy is the first year of life after birth and a newborn child is called an infant from birth till the completion of the first year of life. In the initial half of infancy, the oral cavity has gum pads alone and towards the later half there is the eruption of primary teeth in the oral cavity. Preventive oral care in infancy is the basis of future oral health. The primary aim of a dentist or pediatric dentist at this stage is to educate and motivate the new parents to maintain good oral hygiene of the infant. An infant is completely dependent on the parents/caregivers to fulfil his basic needs. Thus, the entire responsibility of preventive care for optimal oral health lies in the hands of the infant's parents/ caregivers.

1.1. Importance of infant oral health care

Infant oral health is the foundation upon which education and motivation regarding dental hygiene and other preventive dental care must be built on, to augment the prospect of a lifetime free of preventable dental diseases. Infant oral health is an integral part of general well being of an infant, as he or she increases in age. It encompasses the care of the oral cavity and monitoring of the development of the teeth. Unfortunately, pregnant women, parents and caregivers of infants often do not receive timely and accurate education about preventive oral and dental health care [1].

1.2. Role of infant oral health care in preventive dentistry

Prevention is the primary focus of infant oral health care and prevention of dental diseases should be initiated in infancy itself. For diseases that occur early in life such as early childhood caries (ECC) prevention of diseases and the promotion of healthy behavior among parents/ caregivers must be given importance [2]. Preventive oral healthcare must be initiated in infancy because of the following reasons:

1. Poor oral hygiene and improper infant feeding practices create an environment that promotes the colonization of cariogenic bacteria such as *Streptococcus mutans* in the infant's mouth. Thus, when a tooth erupts in an infant's mouth, it is in an undesirable oral environment that promotes demineralization.

2. Risk factors such as improper feeding practices and poor oral hygiene that may lead to early childhood caries (ECC) may be identified at an early age and appropriate intervention may be planned.

3. Parents/caregivers may be educated regarding good oral health care practices to maintain the infant's mouth in a state of good dental health.

4. Undesirable consequences of poor dental health such as ECC may be avoided and the infant may escape its complications such as dental pain and poor nutrition.

5. Psychologic health of the child can be maintained as unesthetic appearance of teeth negatively impacts the psychology of a child.

1.3. Causes and risk factors leading to poor infant oral health

Evidence suggests that early-in-life risk factors play a significant role as predictors of future dental caries in children [3-6]. These risk factors include the extent of parental knowledge, attitude and practices (KAP) and an infant's oral hygiene status, medical history, oral medications and feeding habits. Thus it is important to understand the causes and risk factors of poor infant oral health to avoid the risk of early childhood caries later in life. A major factor contributing to poor infant oral health is insufficient or improper knowledge, attitudes and practices (KAP) related to infant feeding practices and oral care. Evidence gathered from both global and Indian studies shows that both pregnant mothers and parents/caregivers of infants have inadequate KAP regarding infant feeding, weaning, and bottle feeding practices and cleaning of the mouth [7-10]. Lower socio economic status has also been correlated to a low dental KAP [11, 12]. The age group of parents does not show a consistent correlation with lack of dental KAP, with different studies reporting varying results [7, 13]. In addition to the lack of KAP regarding infant oral health, pregnant women seldom attain regular dental care and have dental care needs that are not satisfactorily dealt with [14].

Infants with medically compromised health such as congenital heart disease (CHD) may also be prone to poor oral health. Despite good dental care and intensive prevention, poorer dental health has been seen in children with CHD than in healthy children [15]. Medically compromised children may also have poor oral hygiene since in the presence of life threatening conditions, oral hygiene takes on low priority.

Medical illness and long term medication for it, is another risk factor for poor infant oral health [16-7]. Medically compromised infants are often on long term medication that may have side effects of xerostomia or alteration of salivary properties such as flow, buffering capacity or rate. For example, diuretics are used in congenital heart disease since they increase the excretion of water from the circulatory system. Reduced saliva and altered salivary flow are known side effects of diuretics [18]. Disturbed mineralization in teeth has also been reported

[19]. Additionally, medications in syrup form for infants are often sweetened and this may result in a caries promoting oral environment. Sucrose is still used as a sweetener in some drugs, to enhance flavor [20-1].

Inappropriate infant feeding practices related to bottle feeding, breastfeeding and sweetened pacifiers/ liquids may be another cause of early childhood caries (ECC) as the teeth in the infant [22]. Nighttime bottle feeding with sweetened or sweet liquids is a risk factor for ECC due to salivary reduction and prolonged exposure of the teeth to fermentable carbohydrates [22]. The American Academy of Pediatrics (AAP) recommends breastfeeding as the ideal method of feeding and nurturing infants and recognizes the role of breastfeeding as primary in achieving optimal infant growth and development [23]. Further, the AAP recommends exclusive breastfeeding for the first 6 months followed by the addition of iron-enriched solid foods between 6 to 12 months of age [23]. Though breastfeeding serves several health and immuno-logic advantages to the infant, certain breastfeeding practices may result in ECC. The factors associated with breastfeeding that may result in ECC are ad libitum or at-will feeding, prolonged breastfeeding and frequent breastfeeding during the night, resulting in accumulation of milk in the teeth, which, combined with reduced salivary flow and lack of oral hygiene, may produce tooth decay [24-5].

1.4. Consequences of poor infant oral health

Dental caries remains the most widespread chronic disease of childhood and can have damaging effects on growth and development when it progresses to severe forms [26]. Early childhood caries is a public health problem with its etiologic factors playing a role from infancy itself. Low-income and minority children experience disproportionately more dental caries than other groups because of their added barriers, such as limited access to dental services [27].

Poor infant oral health may lead to early childhood caries which is an infectious disease, and *S. mutans* is the most likely causative agent. Early acquisition, i.e., in infancy, of *S. mutans* is a crucial event in the natural history of ECC [28].

2. The infant's mouth

Oral microbial colonization of an infant's mouth begins shortly after birth [29]. The infants mouth consists only of gum pads in the pre-dentate stage, i.e., till about 6-7 months of age. As the teeth begin to erupt into the oral cavity (as the infant enters dentate stage), the colonization changes as the teeth present additional hard tissue surfaces for colonization. Influences from the mother/caregiver and siblings also play a role in the type of colonization of an infant's mouth.

2.1. Infant Oral Microbiology

The initial microbial microorganisms that colonize an infant's mouth are *Streptococcus salivarius*, *Streptococcus mitis* and *Streptococcus oralis* which belong to the group Mutans streptococcus

[30-3]. Of interest to the dentist is the acquisition of another species of the group Mutans streptococcus – *Streptococcus mutans* (*S. mutans*), which is strongly implicated in the etiology of dental caries [34]. Early-in-life or infant colonization by *S. mutans* is a chief risk factor for early childhood caries and future dental caries [28]. *Streptococcus mutans* was believed to show feeble adhesion to epithelial surfaces found in the pre-dentate infant's mouth [35-6]. The infants' mouth in the pre-dentate stage was thus considered unlikely to harbor *S. mutans* colonization. However, more recent evidence has shown that *S. mutans* colonization does occur in pre-dentate infants and the tongue may serve as an ecological niche in such cases [37-9]. Recently, a new microorganism *Scardovia wiggasiae* has been isolated from the plaque of ECC affected children using polymerase chain reaction (PCR) technology and research in this area is in progress [40].

2.2. Clinical aspects: Acquisition and transmission of *Streptococcus mutans*

Early-in-life acquisition of *Streptococcus mutans* has an impact on the future oral health of infants [28]. Infants may develop oral colonization with *S. mutans* colonization from their colonized parents [41]. The mother is the main source of transmission of S. mutans to a child as seen from clinical and microbiologic studies [42]. Mother-to-child or maternal transmission of *S. mutans* is one of the primary sources of transmission of *S. mutans* to an infant's mouth. This type of transmission of *S. mutans* is also known as *vertical transmission* [43]. In support of this route of transmission, several studies have reported identical bacteriocin profiles [44-5] and plasmid or chromosomal DNA patterns [46-7] of *S. mutans* strains in mother-child pairs. One study reported that when maternal salivary reservoirs exceed 10^5 colony forming units (CFU) the frequency of transmission of *S. mutans* to the infant was 9 times greater than when the maternal salivary levels of *S. mutans* were less than or equal to 10^3 CFU [48].

Horizontal transmission is the other major mode of transmission of *S. mutans* which occurs thorough sharing of spoons, glasses and interpersonal contact between the infant and other members of his/her environment such as siblings, daycare supervisors etc. Evidence for this mode of microbial transmission comes from several studies which have shown that infants and children in the same environment shared *S. mutans* isolates [49, 50]. Accordingly, vertical and horizontal transmission of *S. mutans* needs to be evaluated when taking into account risk factors for dental caries in an infant.

3. Dental home: Concept and advantages

The first step towards promotion of good infant oral health is the creation and maintenance of a dental home. This concept is derived from the concept of medical home that was proposed by the American Academy of Pediatrics in 1992 [51]. The premise behind the medical home was that the best care may be offered to a child when the child in focus and his/her family has a good relationship with the doctor.

The American Academy Pediatric Dentistry (AAPD) recommends that a dental home may be designed for the infant on the same lines as the medical home concept. The characteristics of an ideal dental home are the following [52]:

1. **Accessible:** This implies that dental care should be reachable to the infant and family

2. **Family Centered:** The importance of the family is recognized and behavior management techniques acceptable to the family are utilized.

3. **Continuous:** A dental home should be designed to look after the needs of a child from infancy through adolescence so that continuous care may be provided to the infant at all stages of childhood and adolescence.

4. **Comprehensive:** A dental home provides round-the-clock dental care for a child and includes primary, secondary and tertiary care for the infant.

5. **Coordinated:** An ideal dental home setup works in coordination with school and family of a child so that information may be shared for the benefit of the child in focus.

6. **Compassionate:** In a dental home, good relationships are established with a child's family a community with a concerned and compassionate approach for the child receiving dental care and his/her family.

7. **Culturally Competent:** Since children at a dental home come from varying backgrounds and cultures, an ideal dental home recognizes, values and respects the varied cultures and ethnic backgrounds of children.

There are several advantages of developing a dental home for an infant. Most importantly, the timing of the first dental visit of an infant may be planned within 1 year of age of an infant. This is in accordance with AAPD recommendations for the first dental visit of the child. Early-in-life risk factors can thus be identified at an early stage and appropriate intervention through increase in KAP related to infant feeding and oral hygiene suggested to the parents/caregivers [52]. Moreover, a dental home personalized or tailored preventive program may be designed to suit the specific oral health needs of a child at every stage.

4. Anticipatory guidance

The dental home provides scope for anticipatory guidance at every stage of a child's development. Anticipatory guidance is the process of providing practical, developmentally appropriate information about children's health to prepare parents for the significant physical, emotional and psychological milestones [43, 53]. Anticipatory guidance encompasses 3 types of responsibilities: (1) gathering information, (2) establishing a therapeutic alliance, and (3) providing education and guidance [43, 54].

5. Prenatal oral health counseling

Prenatal oral health counseling for parents is the first step to infant oral healthcare. The rationale of prenatal oral health counseling is to generate awareness among expectant mothers about dental disease, its prevention and the means to promote good oral health in the infant [54]. A mother's DMFS scores, education, and feeding habits are strong risk indicators for the colonization of caries-related micro-organisms and ECC [55].

5.1. Importance of prenatal oral health care (during pregnancy)

Ideally, optimization of infant oral health begins prenatally and continues with the monitoring and counseling of the mother and child, beginning when the infant is approximately 6 months of age, with the eruption of the first tooth [56]. Infants with low birth weight and malnourished infants are at risk for development of enamel hypoplasia [22, 57-8]. Enamel hypoplasia may result in a rough enamel surface which can result in areas more prone to plaque accumulation and resultant caries [57, 59]. Thus, expecting mothers should be advised to optimize nutrition during the third trimester and the infant's first year, when the enamel is undergoing maturation [54]. Recent literature also reports an association between periodontitis in the mother and preterm birth [60] and between *S. mutans* levels in mothers and caries experience in their children [42].

Evaluation of the oral status of expectant mothers followed by pre-and perinatal counseling regarding the expectant mothers' nutrition, oral hygiene, caries experience and KAP regarding infant feeding practices can have a significant impact on the child's caries rate in the future [54]. A dental home can address these needs, if developed at the prenatal stage itself. Pediatric dentists, pediatricians and nutritionists have a combined role in relation to prenatal counseling with a goal to providing the best oral and overall health for the newborn and infant. Future parents should be monitored on a regular basis to ensure effective oral hygiene and dietary habits have been established through regular pre-and perinatal parent counseling.

5.2. Anticipatory guidance for the pregnant mother

Anticipatory guidance has been recommended for the pregnant mother to avoid caries and gingival problems and promote later oral health for the child. These include the following [43, 61-2]:

a.   Education concerning development and prevention of dental disease and also demonstration of oral hygiene procedures.

b.   Counseling to instill preventive attitudes and motivation among mothers.

c.   Providing information to pregnant women about pregnancy gingivitis.

d.   Visiting a dentist for an examination and restoration of all active decay as soon as feasible and to decrease chances of developing pregnancy gingivitis.

e.   Eating healthy foods such as fruits, vegetables, grain products (especially whole grain), and dairy products (milk, cheese) during meals and snacks. Limit eating between meals.

f.   Eating foods containing only sugar at mealtimes, and limiting the amount.

g.   Brushing teeth thoroughly twice a day (after breakfast and before bed) with fluoridated toothpaste and flossing daily.

h.   Rinsing every night with an alcohol-free, over-the-counter fluoridated mouth rinse.

i.   Not smoking cigarettes or chewing tobacco.

6. Infant oral health care: Strategies and methods

An effective approach toward primary prevention of early childhood caries is to develop an approach that targets its infectious element, for example by preventing or delaying primary acquisition of *S. mutans* at an early age or infancy, through suppression of maternal reservoirs of *S. mutans* [63]. Mothers with dense salivary or plaque reservoirs of *S. mutans* are at high risk for transmitting the microorganism to their infants early-in-life [54].

6.1. Parent oral health counseling and education

Parent education and increase in knowledge, attitude and practices (KAP) regarding infant oral health care may provide long lasting benefits on an infant's oral health. Maternal/ Caregiver KAP [7-9] is an area where several lacunae exist regarding infant nutrition, feeding practices and first dental visit. Emphasis must be placed on behavioral approaches to conditions such as ECC that begin early in life the prevention of diseases and the promotion of healthy behavior among mothers and their children [2]. Low-cost health education combined with external motivation proved to be a valuable tool for promoting health behavior in mothers and their children [64].

6.2. Infant feeding related behavior

Infant feeding practices related to breastfeeding, bottle feeding and their timing of cessation must be given importance. Infant formulas are acidogenic and possess cariogenic potential [65-6]. Prenatal and postnatal counseling is essential to generate awareness about the unfavorable consequences of inappropriate infant feeding practices on infant oral health. Recommendations for appropriate infant feeding practices behaviors include [54, 67-8]:

• Infants should not be put to sleep with a bottle containing fermentable carbohydrates.

• At-will breast-feeding should be avoided after the first primary tooth begins to erupt and other dietary carbohydrates are introduced.

• Parents should be encouraged to have infants drink from a cup as they approach their first birthday.

• Infants should be weaned from the bottle at 12 to 14 months of age.

• Repetitive consumption of any liquid containing fermentable carbohydrates from a bottle or training cup should be avoided.

- Between-meal snacks and prolonged exposures to foods and juice or other beverages containing fermentable carbohydrates should be avoided.

6.3. Oral hygiene for the infant

Oral hygiene measures must be implemented no later than the time of eruption of the first primary tooth. These measures include the following [25, 68]:

- If an infant falls asleep while feeding, the teeth should be cleaned before placing the child in bed.

- Tooth brushing of all dentate children should be performed twice daily with a fluoridated toothpaste and a soft, age-appropriate sized toothbrush.

- Parents should use a 'smear' of toothpaste to brush the teeth of a child less than 2 years of age and perform or assist with their child's tooth brushing.

6.4. Fluoride supplementation

Fluoride is a well documented agent in caries control and it may be used for infants also. As per the AAPD, daily fluoride exposure for all children is recommended as a primary preventive procedure [69]. An infant's exposure to drinking water fluoride should be determined based on access to fluoridated water in community water supplies or through water analysis for those drinking well water [69]. A comprehensive knowledge of high fluoride belts and regions with endemic fluorosis is also important especially in countries like India with several geographic high fluoride belts. For infants older than 6 months of age who are exposed to water with less than 0.3 ppm fluoride, dietary fluoride supplements of 0.25 mg fluoride per day should be prescribed [69]. Irrespective of fluoride exposure in water, dietary supplements should not be prescribed for infants under the age of 6 months [69].

7. First dental visit: timing and its relevance

To promote early detection of dental caries and the establishment of a dental home, both the American Academy of Pediatrics (AAP) and American Academy of Pediatric Dentistry recommend the first dental visit by 1 year old. The AAPD recommends that the first oral evaluation visit should occur within 6 months of the eruption of the first primary tooth and no later than 12 months of age [70]. Since *S. mutans* begins to colonize an infant's mouth even prior to tooth eruption, a good dental care regime complemented by a dental home that is established at an initial stage of infancy may lead to long term oral health benefits for the infant.

8. Conclusion

Infant oral health forms the basis of a lifetime of good oral health. The primary focus of infant oral health is prevention and every effort must be made to prevent and promote oral health at this crucial stage of infancy. A dental home must be developed for each child, which provides anticipatory guidance from infancy through adolescence. Maternal education and emphasis on good maternal oral health should also be encouraged at pre-and perinatal stages to further prevent early colonization of cariogenic microorganisms.

Author details

Preetika Chandna* and Vivek K. Adlakha

*Address all correspondence to: drpreetikachandna@gmail.com

Department of Paedodontics and Preventive Dentistry, Subharti Dental College, Meerut, Uttar Pradesh, India

References

[1] Fitzsimons D, Dwyer JT, Palmer C, Boyd LD. Nutrition and oral health guidelines for pregnant women, infants, and children. J Am Diet Assoc. 1998 Feb;98(2):182-6, 189; quiz 187-8.

[2] Hobdell MH, Oliveira ER, Bautista R, Myburgh NG, Lalloo R, Narendran S, Johnson NW. Oral diseases and socioeconomic status (SES). British Dent J 2003:194;91–6.

[3] Alaluusua S, Malmivirta R. Early plaque accumulation: a sign for caries risk in young children. Community Dent Oral Epidemiol. 1994;22:273-6.

[4] Grindefjord M, Dahllof G, Nilsson B, Modeer T. Prediction of dental caries development in 1-year-old children. Caries Res. 1995;29:343-8.

[5] Wendt LK, Hallonsten AL, Koch G, Birkhed D. Analysis of cariesrelated factors in infants and toddlers living in Sweden. Acta Odontol Scand. 1996;54(2):131-7.

[6] Watson MR. Validity of various methods of scoring visible dental plaque as ECC risk measure (abstract 771). J Dent Res. 2001;80:132.

[7] Nagarajappa R, Kakatkar G, Sharda AJ, Asawa K, Ramesh G, Sandesh N. Infant oral health: Knowledge, attitude and practices of parents in Udaipur, India. Dent Res J. 2013;10:659-65.

[8] Nagaraj A, Pareek S. Infant Oral Health Knowledge and Awareness: Disparity among Pregnant Women and Mothers visiting a Government Health Care Organization. Int J Clin Pediatr Dent. 2012;5(3):167-172.

[9] Shivaprakash PK, Elango I, Baweja DK, Noorani HH. The state of infant oral health-care knowledge and awareness: Disparity among parents and healthcare professionals. J Indian Soc Pedod Prev Dent. 2009;27:39-43.

[10] Hoeft KS, Masterson EE, Barker JC. Mexican American mothers' initiation and understanding of home oral hygiene for young children. Pediatr Dent. 2009 Sep-Oct; 31(5):395-404.

[11] Suresh BS, Ravishankar TL, Chaitra TR, Mohapatra AK, Gupta V. Mother's knowledge about pre-school child's oral health. J Indian Soc Pedod Prev Dent. 2010;28:282-7.

[12] Williams NJ, Whittle JG, Gatrell AC. The relationship between socio-demographic characteristics and dental health knowledge and attitudes of parents with young children. Br Dent J 2002;193:651-4.

[13] Rwakatema DS, Ng'ang'a PM. Oral health knowledge, attitudes and practices of parents/guardians of pre-school children in Moshi, Tanzania. East Afr Med J 2009;86:520-5.

[14] Villa A, Abati S, Pileri P, Calabrese S, Capobianco G, Strohmenger L, Ottolenghi L, Cetin I, Campus GG. Oral health and oral diseases in pregnancy: a multicentre survey of Italian postpartum women. Aust Dent J. 2013 Jun;58(2):224-9.

[15] Stecksen-Blicks C, Rydberg A, Nyman L, Asplund S, Svanberg C. Dental car-ies experience in children with congenital heart disease: a case-control study. Int J Paediatr Dent 2004;14:94-100.

[16] Moore PA, Guggenheimer J. Medication-induced hyposalivation: etiology, diagnosis, and treatment. Compend Contin Educ Dent. 2008;29:50-5.

[17] Maupome G, Shulman JD, Medina-Solis CE, Ladeinde O. Is there a relation-ship between asthma and dental caries?: a critical review of the literature. J Am Dent Assoc. 2010;141:1061-74.

[18] Scully C, Felix DH. Oral medicine-update for the dental practitioner lumps and swellings. Br Dent J. 2005;199:763-70.

[19] Hakala PE, Haavikko K. Permanent tooth formation of children with congenital cyanotic heart disease. Proc Finn Dent Soc 1974;70:63-6.

[20] Bigeard L. The role of medication and sugars in Paediatric dental patients. Dent Clin North Am. 2000; 44:443-56.

[21] Moursi AM, Fernandez JB, Daronch M, Zee L, Jones CL. Nutrition and oral health considerations in children with special health care needs: implications for oral health care providers. Pediatr Dent. 2010; 32:333-42.

[22] Seow WK. Biological mechanisms of early childhood caries. Community Dent Oral Epidemiol. 1998; 26 (1 Suppl):8-27.

[23]   Breastfeeding and the use of human milk. Pediatrics. 2012 Mar;129(3):e827-41.

[24]   Schafer TE, Adair SM. Prevention of dental disease. Pediatr Clin North Am. 2000;47:1021-42

[25]   McDonald R, Avery D, Dean J Mosby. Dentistry for the Child and the Adolescent. 8th Ed St. Louis, Missouri: Mosby; 2004.

[26]   Dela Cruz GG, Rozier G, Slade G. Dental screening and referral of young children by pediatric primary care providers. Pediatrics. 2006;114:642-52.

[27]   Lewis CW, Grossman DC, Domoto PK, Deyo RA. The role of the pediatrician in the oral health of children: A national survey. Pediatrics. 2002;106:84-90.

[28]   Berkowitz RJ. Causes, treatment and prevention of early childhood caries: a micro-biologic perspective. J Can Dent Assoc. 2003 May;69(5):304-7.

[29]   Law V, Seow WK, Townsend G. Factors influencing oral colonization of mutans streptococci in young children. Aust Dent J. 2007 Jun;52(2):93-100; quiz 159.

[30]   Pearce C, Bowden GH, Evans M, et al. Identification of pioneer viridans streptococci in the oral cavity of human neonates. J Med Microbiol. 1995;42:67-72.

[31]   Kononen E, Asikainen S, Saarela M, Karjalainen J, Jousimies-Somer H. The oral gram-negative anaerobic microflora in young children: longitudinal changes from edentulous to dentate mouth. Oral Microbiol Immunol. 1994;9:136-41.

[32]   Rotimi VO, Duerden BI. The development of the bacterial flora in normal neonates. J Med Microbiol. 1981;14:51-62.

[33]   Carlsson J, Grahnen H, Jonsson G. Lactobacilli and streptococci in the mouth of children. Caries Res. 1975;9:333-9.

[34]   van Houte J. Role of micro-organisms in caries etiology. J Dent Res 1994;73:672-681.

[35]   Gibbons RJ. Bacteriology of dental caries. J Dent Res. 1964;43:1021–8.

[36]   Gibbons RJ, Houte JV. Bacterial adherence in oral microbial ecology. Annu Rev Microbiol. 1975;29:19–44.

[37]   Wan AK, Seow WK, Purdie DM, Bird PS, Walsh LJ, Tudehope DI. Oral colonization of *Streptococcus mutans* in six-month-old predentate infants. *J Dent Res* 2001; 80(12): 2060–5.

[38]   Ramos-Gomez FJ, Weintraub JA, Gansky SA, Hoover CI, Featherstone JD. Bacterial, behavioral and environmental factors associated with early childhood caries. J Clin Pediatr Dent 2002; 26(2):165–73.

[39]   Tanner AC, Milgrom PM, Kent R Jr, Mokeem SA, Page RC, Riedy CA, Weinstein P, Bruss J. The microbiota of young children from tooth and tongue samples. J Dent Res. 2002 Jan;81(1):53-7.

[40] Tanner AC, Mathney JM, Kent RL, Chalmers NI, Hughes CV, Loo CY, Pradhan N, Kanasi E, Hwang J, Dahlan MA, Papadopolou E, Dewhirst FE Cultivable anaerobic microbiota of severe early childhood caries. J Clin Microbiol. 2011 Apr;49(4):1464-74.

[41] Douglass JM, Li Y, Tinanoff N. Association of mutans streptococci between caregivers and their children. Pediatr Dent 2008; 30:375-87.

[42] Berkowitz R. Mutans streptococci: Acquisition and transmission. Pediatr Dent. 2006;28:106-9.

[43] Pinkham J, Casamassimo P, Fields H, McTigue D, Nowak A. Pediatric Dentistry: Infancy through Adolescence. 4th Ed. Philadelphia: Saunders; 2005.

[44] Berkowitz RJ, Jordan H. Similarity of bacteriocins and Streptotoccus mutans from mother and infant. Arch Oral Biol. 1975; 20(11):725–30.

[45] Davey AL, Rogers AH. Multiple types of the bacterium *Streptococcus mutans* in the human mouth and their intra-family transmission. Arch Oral Biol. 1984; 29(6):453–60.

[46] Caufield PW, Wannemuehler Y, Hensen J. Familiar clustering of the *Streptococcus mutans* cryptic plasmid strain in a dental clinic population. Infect Immun. 1982; 38(2): 785–7.

[47] Kulkarni GV, Chan KH, Sandham HJ. An investigation into the use of restriction endonuclease analysis in the study of transmission of mutans streptococci. J Dent Res. 1989; 68(7):1155–61

[48] Berkowitz RJ, Turner J, Green P. Maternal salivary levels of *Streptococcus mutans* and primary oral infection in infants. Arch Oral Biol 1981; 26(2):147–9.

[49] Mattos-Graner RO, Smith DJ, King WF, Mayer MP. Water insoluble glucan synthesis by mutans streptococcal strains correlates with caries incidence in 12-to 30-month-old children. J Dent Res. 2000;79:1371-7.

[50] van Loveren C, Buijs JF, ten Cate JM. Similarity of bacteriocin activity profiles of mutans streptococci within the family when the children acquire the strains after the age of 5. Caries Res 2000; 34(6):481–5.

[51] The American Academy of Pediatrics Ad Hoc Task Force on Definition of the Medical Home. The medical home. Pediatr. 1992;90:774.

[52] Nowak AJ, Casamassimo PS. The dental home: a primary care oral health concept. J Am Dent Assoc. 2002 Jan;133(1):93-8.

[53] Lewis CW, Grossman DC, Domoto PK, Deyo RA. The role of the pediatrician in the oral health of children: A National survey. Pediatr. 2000;106:E84.

[54] Chandna P, Adlakha VK. Oral health in children guidelines for pediatricians. Indian Pediatr. 2010 Apr;47(4):323-7.

[55] Ersin NK, Eronat N, Cogulu D, Uzel A, Aksit S. Association of maternal-child charac-teristics as a factor in early childhood caries and salivary bacterial counts. J Dent Child (Chic). 2006 May-Aug;73(2):105-11.

[56] Gomez SS, Weber AA. Effectiveness of a caries preventive program in pregnant women and new mothers on their offspring. Int J Paediatr Dent. 2001;11:117-22.

[57] Seow WK, Humphrys C, Tudehope DI. Increased prevalence of developmental den-tal defects in low birth-weight, prematurely born children: a controlled study. Pe-diatr Dent. 1987;9:221-5.

[58] Davies GN. Early childhood caries–a synopsis. Community Dent Oral Epidemiol 1998;26(1 Suppl):106-16.

[59] Horowitz HS. Research issues in early childhood caries. Community Dent Oral Epi-demiol 1998;26(1 Suppl):67-81.

[60] McGaw T. Periodontal disease and preterm delivery of low-birth-weight infants. J Can Dent Assoc. 2002;68:165-9.

[61] Brambilla E, Felloni A, Gagliani M, Malerba A, García-Godoy F, Strohmenger L. Ca-ries prevention during pregnancy: results of a 30-month study. J Am Dent Assoc. 1998;129:871-7.

[62] Nowak AJ, Casamassimo PS. Using anticipatory guidance to provide early dental in-tervention. J Am Dent Assoc. 1995;126:1156-63.

[63] Kohler B, Bratthall D, Krasse B. Preventive measures in mothers influence the estab-lishment of the bacterium *Streptococcus mutans* in their infants. *Arch Oral Biol* 1983; 28(3):225–31.

[64] Mohebbia SZ, Virtanen JI, Vehkalahtic MM. Improvements in the Behaviour of Mother-Child Pairs Following Low-cost Oral Health Education. Oral Health Prev Dent 2014;1:13-1.

[65] Sheikh C, Erickson PR. Evaluation of plaque pH changes following oral rinse with eight infant formulas. Pediatr Dent. 1996;18:200-4.

[66] Bowen WH, Pearson SK, Rosalen PL, Miguel JC, Shih AY. Assessing the cariogenic potential of some infant formulas, milk and sugar solutions. J Am Dent Assoc. 1997;128:865-71.

[67] American Academy on Pediatric Dentistry Council on Clinical Affairs. Policy on ear-ly childhood caries (ECC): unique challenges and treatment option. Pediatr Dent. 2008-2009;30(7 Suppl):44-6.

[68] American Academy on Pediatric Dentistry Council on Clinical Affairs. Policy on ear-ly childhood caries (ECC): classifications, consequences, and preventive strategies. Pediatr Dent. 2008-2009;30(7 Suppl):40-3.

[69] American Academy on Pediatric Dentistry Liaison with Other Groups Committee; American Academy on Pediatric Dentistry Council on Clinical Affairs. Guideline on fluoride therapy. Pediatr Dent. 2008-2009;30(7 Suppl):121-4.

[70] American Academy of Pediatric Dentistry. Clinical Affairs Committee-Infant Oral Health Subcommittee. Guideline on infant oral health care. Pediatr Dent. 2012 Sep-Oct;34(5):148-52

7

Fissure Sealing in Occlusal Caries Prevention

Kristina Goršeta

1. Introduction

In the modern world there is still a problem of dental caries. Dental caries is still the most common chronic childhood disease and the primary cause of tooth loss. Over the past 30 years, significant progress has been made in the prevention of dental caries in children and adolescents. While caries has decreased on interproximal surfaces, occlusal pit and fissure caries have increased [1, 2]. In general, research has demonstrated that caries on occlusal and buccal/lingual surfaces account for almost 90% of caries experienced in children and adolescents [3]. The caries process in the first and second molars usually starts soon after eruption. The occlusal surfaces of lateral teeth, especially molars have complicated morphology with many grooves (fissures) and pits on the occlusal surface and on the buccal and palatal surfaces (Figure 1). These molar teeth are considered the most susceptible teeth to dental caries due to the anatomy of the chewing surfaces of these teeth, which unfortunately inhibits protection from saliva and fluoride and instead favours plaque accumulation [4]. Pits and fissures don't cause caries process. They permit the entrance of microorganisms and food into this sheltered warm moist richly provided incubator and the dental plaque can be expected to form here. They instead provide a sanctuary to those agents, which cause caries. When carbohydrates in food come in contact with the plaque, acidogenic bacteria in the plaque create acid. This acid damages the enamel walls of the pits and fissures and caries results. Therefore, the most decay is concentrated on the occlusal surfaces of posterior molars.

Pits and fissures have variations in their appearance in cross section. They were described based on the alphabetical description of shape. According to Nango (1960) there were 4 types of pits and fissures: V&U type: self cleansing and somewhat caries resistant; U type: narrow slit like opening with a larger base-susceptible to caries and a number of different ranches K type: also very susceptible to caries [5]. These are the sites most susceptible to developing decay [6].

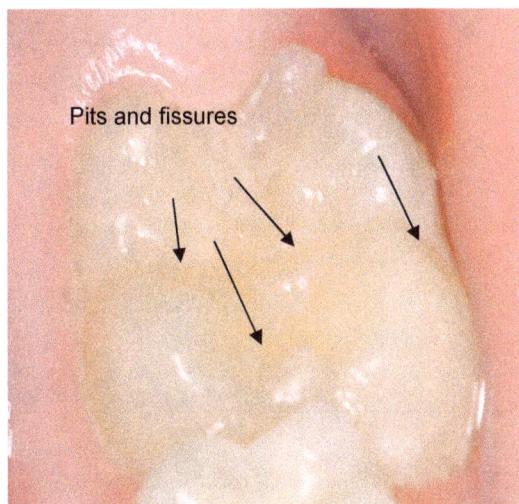

Figure 1. Occlusal morphology of molar teeth

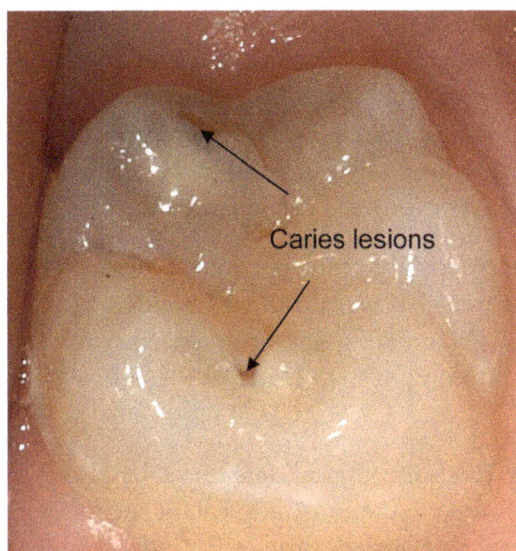

Figure 2. Caries lesions on the occlusal surface of molar tooth

In most cases the shape of the pit or fissure is such that it is impossible to clean, explaining the high susceptibility of pits and fissures to dental caries (Figure 2 and 3). Caries in the pits and fissures follows the direction of enamel rods and characteristically forms a triangular or cone shaped lesion with its apex at the outer surface and its base towards DEJ. Pits and fissures provide greater cavitations than smooth surface caries. Preventive measures for tooth decay include daily tooth brushing, topical fluoride application, chewing gums with xylitol and sealing of fissures which are applied by dental clinicians [7-10].

There have been many efforts made within past decades to prevent the development of caries, in particular occlusal caries as it was once generally accepted that pits and fissures of teeth

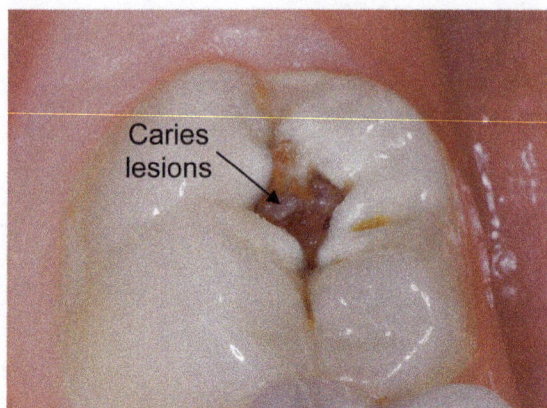

Figure 3. Caries lesion in the fissure of molar tooth

would become infected with bacteria within 10 years of erupting into the mouth [7-10]. G.V. Black, the creator of modern dentistry, informed that more than 40% of caries incidences in permanent teeth occurred in pits and fissures due to being able to retain food and plaque [9].There were many attempts to prevent occlusal caries. Willoughby D. Miller, a pioneer of dentistry, was applying silver nitrate with its antibacterial functions to surfaces of teeth to prevent occlusal caries in early 1905. It was chemically treating the biofilm against both Streptococcus mutans and Actinomyces naeslundii, which are both carious pathogens [7-9, 11]. Silver nitrate, which was also being practiced by H. Klein and J.W. Knutson in the 1940s, was being used in attempt to prevent and arrest occlusal caries [9,12].

In 1955, M.G. Buonocore gave insight to the benefits of etching enamel with phosphoric acid. [7-9] His studies demonstrated that resin could be bonded to enamel through acid etching, increasing adhesion whilst also creating an improved marginal integrity of resin restorative material [7,9]. Later, this bonding system leads to the future successful creation of fissure sealants [8-13].

By the late 1970s and early 1980s the clinical data on sealants and caries prevention was very positive. Studies have continued to demonstrate sealant success. One 4-year study showed an overall 43% decrease in the prevalence of caries effectiveness with significantly better sealant retention on premolars (84%) than molars (30%) [5]. A 7-year study reported 66% complete sealant retention and 14% partial retention [9]. Sealant loss was 20% while there was a 55% reduction in caries rate for the sealed teeth versus the unsealed teeth. One 10-year study showed that for over 8,000 sealants placed on permanent first molars, there was 41% complete sealant retention at 10 years and a 58%–63% retention rate over 7 to 9 years [10].

2. Sealants materials

Pit and fissure sealants proved to be an effective clinical intervention to prevent occlusal caries [13-15]. The aim of fissure sealants is to prevent or arrest the development of dental caries [15].

Preventing tooth decay from the pits and fissures of the teeth is achieved by the fissure sealants blocking these surfaces and therefore stopping food and bacteria from getting stuck in these grooves and fissures [15]. Fissure sealants also provide a smooth surface that is easily accessible for both our natural protective factor, saliva and the toothbrush bristles when cleaning our teeth. Fissure sealing prevents the growth of bacteria in fissures that cause tooth decay. There are several types of materials for fissure sealing.

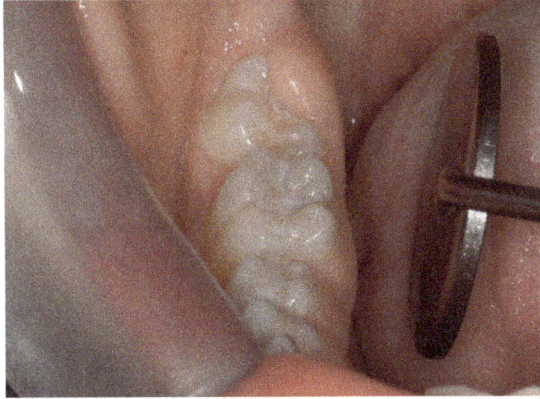

Figure 4. Fissure sealed with resin based sealant material

Caries in pits and fissures has responded less to routine preventive methods than caries on smooth surfaces. Pit and fissure sealant use is an effective clinical regime available for preventing occlusal caries. The most widely used pit and fissure sealants are based on bis-glycidyl methacrylate (Bis-GMA) resins. These resins were introduced in 1963 as restorative materials. The main types in use are resin-based sealants and glass ionomer cements [16, 17]. Cueto and Buonocore suggested the sealing of pits and fissures with an adhesive resin in 1967 [18,19]. E.I. Cueto created the first sealant material, which was methyl cyanoacrylate [7, 11,19]. However, this material was susceptible to bacterial breakdown over time, therefore was not an acceptable sealing material [18]. Bunonocore made further advances in 1970 by developing bisphenol-a glycidyl dimethacrylate, which is a viscous resin commonly known as BIS-GMA [13]. This material was used as the basis for many resin-based sealant/composite material developments in dentistry, as it is resistant to bacterial breakdown and forms a steady bond with etched enamel [13,19, 30].

A second group of materials used as fissure sealants are the glass ionomer cements (Figure 5). Glass ionomer cement is also the material of choice for fissure sealing. In 1974, glass ionomer cement fissure sealants (GIC) were introduced by J.W. McLean and A.D. Wilson [15,38]. GIC materials bond both to enamel and dentine after being cleaned with polyacrylic acid conditioner [15]. Some other advantages GIC's have is that they contain fluoride and are less moisture sensitive, with suggestions being made that despite having poor retention, they may prevent occlusal caries even after the sealant has fallen out due to their ability to release fluoride[7,13,14-16].

It has certain advantages over composite resins: less susceptible to moisture, easy handling and long-term release of fluoride ions [20,21]. These are all essential characteristics for materials handled in paediatric dentistry. However, various studies have shown a significantly lower level of retention compared with composite resins [22-25]. Mechanical properties of glass ionomer are significantly weaker than composite resin. Question about preventive effect of glass ionomer still gets controversial answers: Different studies have shown different preventive effects [22, 24, 21,26, 27].

Glass ionomer materials release fluoride over time and have the advantage of being less sensitive to moisture contamination than resin-based materials, making them a potential alternative to resin-based sealants when moisture control is an issue [28,29]. Hybrid materials which incorporate features of both resin and glass ionomer, e.g. polyacid-modified resins (compomers) and resin-modified glass ionomers, have also been developed and used as pit and fissure sealants [30].

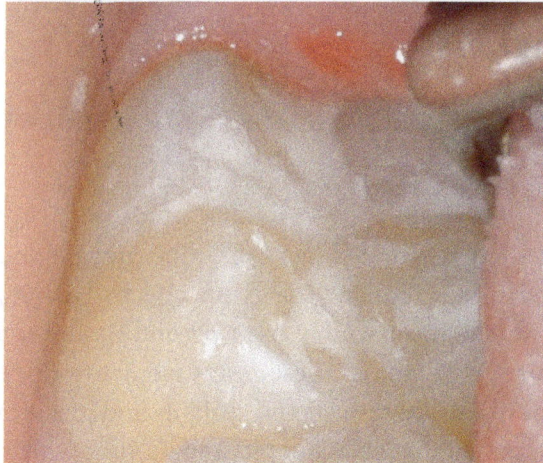

Figure 5. Fissure sealed with glass ionomer sealant material

3. Properties of fissure sealing materials

Resin-based fissure sealants are effective at preventing caries on pit and fissure surfaces in children and adolescents. A Cochrane systematic review of 16 trials found that first permanent molar teeth sealed with resin-based sealant had 78% less caries on occlusal surfaces after 2 years and 60% less after 4–4.5 years compared to unsealed molars [31]. Sealant retention is critical to the effectiveness of resin-based sealants and retention has become an important measure of sealant effectiveness. The Cochrane systematic review reported complete sealant retention rates and it ranged from 79% to 92% at 12 months, 71% to 85% at 24 months, 61% to 80% at 36 months, 52% at 48 months, 72% at 54 months and 39% at 9 years [31]. There was evidence of a clear trend for decreasing sealant retention with time. Some other systematic review on sealant effectiveness reported that the caries-preventive effect of sealants was influenced by sealant replacement, with relatively high reductions in caries risk found in those studies in which a sealant replacement strategy had been used [32].

To achieve effective caries prevention on occlusal surfaces, dental sealants should have several properties. Adhesion of material should be perfect during all kind of function and thermal challenges. Dimensional changes of material during setting should be minimal. Complete retention of sealant material in the occlusal fissures depends on the dimensional changes and resistance to wear and fracture. Good preventive effect today means substantial release of fluoride ions.

Glass ionomer cements (GICs) are also proposed for pit and fissure sealant materials. They have several advantages compared to classic resin sealant materials: easy handling, fluoride releasing at a continuous rate and they are not moisture sensitive.

For the best caries preventive effect in the fissures of lateral teeth, material for sealing should have the following properties:

1. Ideal adhesion of material should be maintained during setting and function, including the challenges of both thermal and mechanical cycling.

2. Complete retention of the sealant material in the occlusal fissures

3. Resistance to wear and fracture

4. Ease to handling and placement

5. Caries preventive effects

6. Biocompatibility.

Inclusion of fluoride ions in the material may be beneficial on the prevention of developing carious lesions, and the remineralization of any demineralized enamel adjacent to the sealant [33-37].

Some studies introduced additional treatment to improve mechanical properties of glass ionomer materials. So a few years ago a method of heating the glass ionomer was introduced. Material was heated with 60-70oC metal plates in order to improve the mechanical properties of materials [39]. Sidhu and colleagues have linked the contraction of the material and the loss of water from glass ionomer cement as a reason to improve the properties of materials[40]. Some studies have shown enhanced adhesion of glass ionomer for hard tissues [95].

Another study tried to increase the level of retention of glass ionomer sealants with heating during setting time of materials [41]. The results obtained for the resin sealing group as a control group in this study are consistent with previously published studies and their results [41-44]. Glass ionomer (Fuji VII) on the basis of the results obtained by monitoring of patient showed a relatively low percentage of retention after 12 months. The results did not differ when compared with the results obtained for the retention of classical (chemical) treated glass ionomer cement [45-50].

4. Caries preventive effect

There is good evidence that teeth sealed very early after eruption require more frequent reapplication of the FS than teeth sealed later [51,52]. Therefore, FS placement may be delayed until the teeth are fully erupted, unless high caries activity is present. Placement of FS even in the absence of regular follow-up is beneficial [53, 54].

Caries prevalence is relatively low in high-income and relatively high in low-and middle-income countries. Children from high-income countries have benefited from the available established caries preventive measures; such as the use of fluoride-containing products and awareness among their parents and caretakers of the importance of keeping tooth surfaces free from plaque [55].

The studies show that sealants work if applied correctly. Sealant success is multifactorial [56, 57]. Technique, fissure morphology, and the characteristics of the sealant contribute to clinical success [58]. When one reviews published sealant data, a basic concept of 5%–10% of sealant loss per year has been seen demonstrated [31, 32]. This data reveal the importance of re-evaluating teeth with sealants on a periodic basis and to reapply if necessary.

Discussion about caries preventive effect of glass ionomer sealants is still controversial: different studies have shown different preventive effects. It was reported that some material remnants in the fissures can maintain caries prevention. The treatment of glass ionomer material with thermo-curing was recently introduced and showed increase of the mechanical properties. Gorseta et al. showed increased bond strength of glass ionomers to hard dental tissues after thermo-curing during material setting [58]. Skrinjaric et al. investigated the retention rate of glass ionomer sealant material thermo-cured during setting time after 1-year clinical trial [41]. Some authors have pointed to the fact that the remains of SIC in the fissures may have some preventive effect in the development of caries [59, 60]. Skrinjaric et al. did not determine SIC remains in fissures. Increased cariostatic effect can be achieved by regular reapplication, but it increases the cost of such preventing procedure [61-64]. The Database Cochane Review could not find a conclusion on a comparison of glass ionomer sealants and resin sealants [63]. Therefore, it is an area that needs further investigation in order to obtain relevant conclusions.

Primary objective of the most studies is to evaluate the effectiveness of pit and fissure sealants in children and adolescents. It is very important that a different background level of caries in the population is related to obtained results. The diagnosis of the surface to be sealed was based on clinical examination in nine studies, one further study used also a DIAGNOdent device [65-68].

Studies which compare the retention of two or more nearly similar type of sealant materials and report the caries rates only on the sealed occlusal surfaces are not relevant. It is important to report on individual level. Information on the caries risk in the study population, the use of fluoridated water, toothpaste and general preventive methods as well as other preventive interventions should be reported in order to facilitate multivariate analysis of risk factors [69].

Comparing glass ionomers to resin sealants, where less than 10% of tooth surfaces had a small dentine caries lesion and most tooth surfaces were reported to be sound. Caries diagnosis of occlusal surfaces can be challenging. In general, using conventional visual, tactile and radiographic methods in occlusal caries lesion diagnosis, it is not accurate enough to identify whether a lesion extends into the dentine or not [70].

New technologies such as DIAGNOdent laser fluorescence devices may be more sensitive in detecting occlusal dentinal caries [71, 72]. However, the likelihood of false-positive diagnoses may increase when using laser-fluorescence compared with visual methods [71]. Regardless of the caries diagnostic method used, the condition of an occlusal surface to be sealed remains, however, in any case somewhat unclear.

5. Indications and contraindications

Post eruption period of the tooth is most caries susceptible. According to EAPD guidelines, fissure sealant should be placed as soon as possible if there is an indication for placement. However, teeth can be sealed at any age depending on assessment of caries risk factors. [15].

Indications for the use of dental sealants are individual and it depends on patients or teeth that are at high risk of dental caries.

This includes patients with:

- Patients with high risk of dental caries

- Poor oral hygiene

- Deep pits and fissures

- Enamel defects or hypomineralisation or hypoplasia

- Initial lesion of dental caries

- Orthodontics appliances.[73]

Contraindications for the use of dental sealants are individual patients or teeth that are at a low risk of dental caries:

This includes patients with:

- Teeth with shallow, self-cleansing fissures

- Adequate oral hygiene

- A balanced diet with low carbohydrates intake

- Partially erupted teeth without adequate moisture control (operators may choose to use GIC in these cases)

- Teeth with previously restored pits and fissures.[73]

6. Clinical procedure for fissure sealing

It includes:

1. **Tooth selection** (Figure 6) and cleaning the occlusal surface (Figure 7).

Visual dental examination is the starting point for dental assessment and treatment planning. The assessment of occlusal surfaces is particularly challenging, due to their complex morphology. The basic prerequisites for visual caries detection are clean, dry teeth and good illumination [72, 74, 75].

The difficulty in detecting and correctly assessing occlusal caries by visual examination alone has led to the development of various caries detection methods to refine the diagnostic process, and to enhance the identification of early caries lesions [68, 71, 73]. These methods include dental radiography, light-based technologies e.g. fibre-optic transillumination, quantitative laser fluorescence (DIAGNOdent) or light induced fluorescence (QLF). Given the importance of the visual examination, a system for detailed visual examination of teeth – the International Caries Detection and Assessment System (ICDAS) – has been developed, which promotes the recording of the earliest changes in enamel as well as dentinal caries [76].

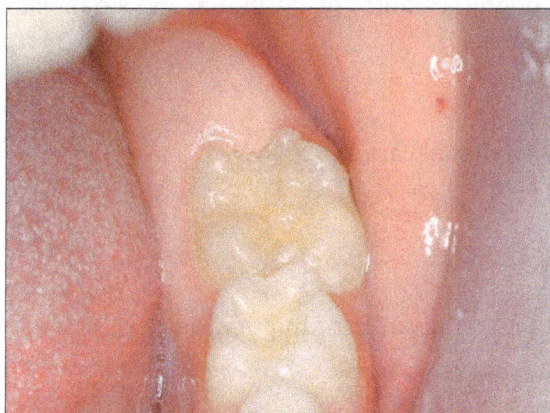

Figure 6. Tooth selected for sealing

There are different approaches for surface cleaning and the way of cleaning pits and fissures before sealing. It may seem to be controversial. Raadal et al. suggested careful removal of pellicle and plaque with pumice in order to achieve optimal acid-etch pattern of the enamel [77]. On the other hand, Harris and Garcia-Godoy keep that the enamel acid etching alone is sufficient for surface cleaning and provided soft plaque removal [78]. The literature is extensive on the effectiveness of different methods for cleaning prior to bonding [15]. Air abrasion also has been suggested for preparation of the occlusal surface before sealant application [79]. In this case a high-speed stream of purified aluminium oxide particles propelled by air pressure is used to clean the tooth surface. They can remove debris and excavate incipient decay in the fissures. A widening of the fissures with rotary instrumentation in order to remove superficial enamel and open the fissure to have the resin penetrate into it has been recommended before

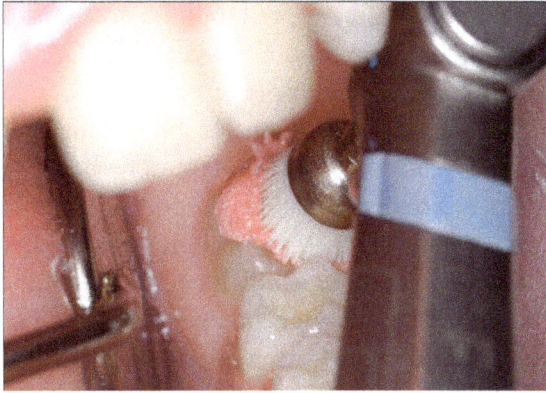

Figure 7. Cleaning the occlusal surface

etching and sealant application by Waggoner and Siegal. This is known as the invasive pit-and fissure technique [80, 81]. However, although cleaning the fissures with a bur has given superior retention in some studies [82, 83]. There is evidence in other studies that it provides no additional benefit [84]. Furthermore, purpose full removal of enamel or enameloplasty just to widen the base of a fissure in a sound occlusal surface is an invasive technique, which disturbs the equilibrium of the fissure system and exposes a child unnecessarily to the use of a handpiece or air abrasion. It is concluded, therefore, that there is a need for removal of most organic substance in order to obtain sufficient bonding, but that the removal of sound tooth tissue by the use of instruments, such as a bur, is unnecessary and undesirable. There is a significant volume of evidence of high fissure sealants retention without the use of a bur. Hydrogen peroxide (3%) also has been suggested for cleaning the occlusal fissures before etching, but there is no evidence that this improves clinical retention [85].

2.   Moisture control

Adequate isolation is the most critical aspect of the sealant application process [78]. Achieving good moisture control is one of the greatest challenges to successful sealant application. Salivary contamination of a tooth surface during or after acid etching will have a key effect on the bond quality between enamel and resin. Salivary contamination, also allows the precipitation of glycoprotein onto the enamel surface greatly decreasing bond strength. If the enamel porosity created by the etching procedure is filled by any kind of liquid, the formation of resin tags in the enamel is blocked or reduced [86, 87]. The circumstances that affect the control of moisture will vary from patient to patient, and may relate to the state of eruption of the tooth, the patient's ability to co-operate, the materials and equipment available for isolation, or a combination of these factors. The options considered by the Guideline Group for 'interim' treatment of teeth for which a sealant was indicated but for which adequate isolation could not be achieved were: resin-based sealant, fluoride varnish and glass ionomer sealant [15].

The rubber dam, when properly placed, provides the best, the safest way of moisture control, and for an operator working alone, it ensures properly isolation from start to finish. In young and partially erupted teeth this is usually not practical. There is evidence of difficulty in securely placing a clamp onto a partially erupted tooth, discomfort during clamp placement and it demands the use of local analgesia in some instances [7, 15]. On the other hand, there is sufficient evidence that careful isolation with cotton rolls gives similar retention results [83]. Cotton roll isolation offers some advantages over rubber dam isolation. No anaesthetic is necessary because no clamps are placed. Cotton rolls can be held in place with either cotton roll holders or fingers. The primary disadvantage to cotton roll isolation is that it is almost a practical necessity that an assistant be used to provide four-handed dentistry [88-90]. The maintenance of a dry field must therefore usually be achieved by the use of cotton rolls and isolation shields, in combination with a thoughtful use of the water spray and evacuation tip. The isolation procedure may frequently be extremely challenging, particularly in the partially erupted teeth or in those children with poor cooperation.

3.   Enamel cleaning(Figure 8)

The goal of etching is to produce a dry, uncontaminated and frosted surface [91]. There are various etching materials available, but the most frequently used is orthophosphoric acid, provided that its concentration lies between 30% and 50% by weight. This is available as both a liquid solution and a gel. Small variations in the concentration do not appear to affect the quality of the etched surface [81]. Duggal et al. showed no significant difference in retention of fissure sealant after one year follow-up on second primary and first permanent molars when 15, 30, 45 or 60 seconds etching times were used [92]. Liquid etching, likewise, is often applied by brush or a small cotton pledget. The application of the gel is often done either directly from the gel dispenser with special applicator tips or with a small disposable brush [7].

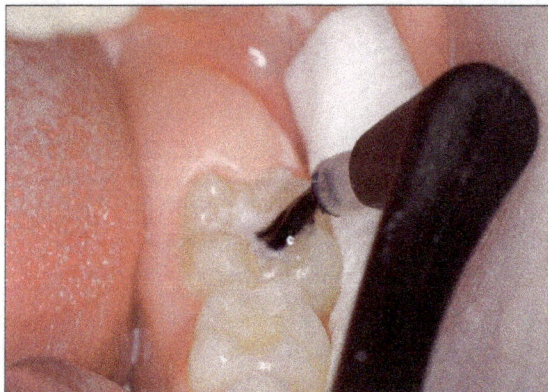

Figure 8. Etching the occlusal surface

4.   Rinsing and drying

Many of the sealant manufacturers recommend rinsing the tooth for 20 to 30 seconds to remove the etchant. The most important is ensuring that the rinse is long enough to remove all of the etchant from the surface. After drying the tooth with compressed air, the tooth exhibits a chalky, frosted appearance but if still no milky white appearance is seen, the tooth should be re-etched for 15 to 20 seconds [7, 81, 91].

5. Sealant application (Figure 9)

During sealant application, all the susceptible pits and fissures should be sealed for maximum caries protection. The long-term clinical success of fissure sealants is closely related to their poor handling [93]. The sealant material can be applied to the tooth in a variety of methods. It may be applied with a small brush or on the tip of an explorer. Some common problems occur during sealant application. Small bubbles may form in the sealant material. If these are present, they should be teased out with a brush before polymerization. Many sealant kits have their own dispensers, which directly apply the sealant to the tooth surface. When using a dispenser, the dentist should allow the sealant to flow ahead into the pits and fissures. It reduces air entrapment [7].

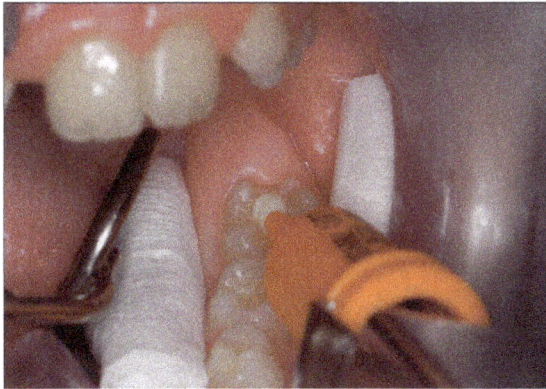

Figure 9. Application of glass ionomer fissure sealing material

6. Application of surface gloss for glass ionomer sealants (Figure 10)

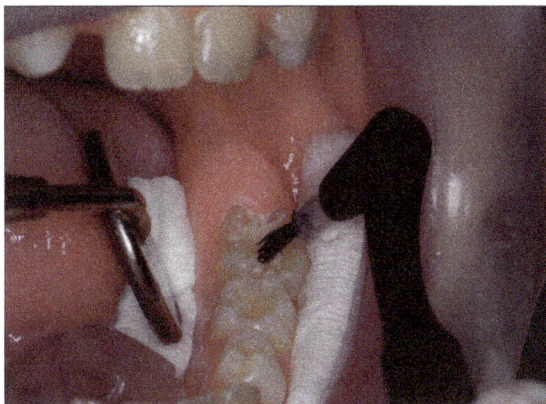

Figure 10. Application of surface gloss

7.   Polymerization of resin sealants or Thermo-curing of glass ionomer sealants (Figure 11)

For light cured sealants, polymerization should be initiated quickly after the sealant is placed on the etched surface to help minimize potential contamination. Some study found that the longer sealants were allowed to sit on the etched surface before being polymerized; the more the sealant penetrated the microporosities, creating longer resin tags, which are critical for micromechanical retention [94]. One of the key factors affecting polymerisation is the light intensity of the dental light curing unit. A Canadian study reported that 12.1% of light curing units tested in a sample of dental practices had intensities that would be considered inadequate (<300 mW/cm²) [70]. Other factors that may influence polymerisation include curing time, distance of the light guide from the material being cured, and thickness, shade and composition of the material being cured.

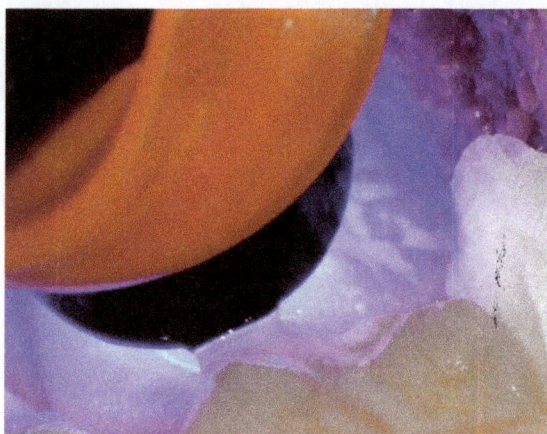

Figure 11. Thermo-curing with dental light

There are some tips for better fissure sealants:

a.   Cure each surface on the same tooth separately if more than one surface is being sealed

b.   Put the light-curing tip as close as possible to the surface and cure for at least the recommended curing time.

c.   Manufacturer's instructions for sealant materials and for curing lights should be available for every operator

d.   Check the light output and curing performance of dental curing units in accordance with the manufacturer's instructions

8.   Evaluation of the sealed tooth (Figure 12)

Sealant retention should be checked with a probe after application, and the sealant re-applied, if necessary, repeating each step of the sealant application procedure.

Regular evaluation of sealants for retention is critical to their success. During routine recall examinations, it is necessary to re-evaluate the sealed tooth surface both visually and tactually for loss of material, exposure of voids in the material and caries development. The need for reapplication of sealants is usually highest during the first six months after placement [95]. When sealants are partially lost and require repair, the clinician should vigorously attempt to dislodge the remaining sealant material with an explorer. If it remains intact to probing, there is no need to completely remove the old material before placing the new.

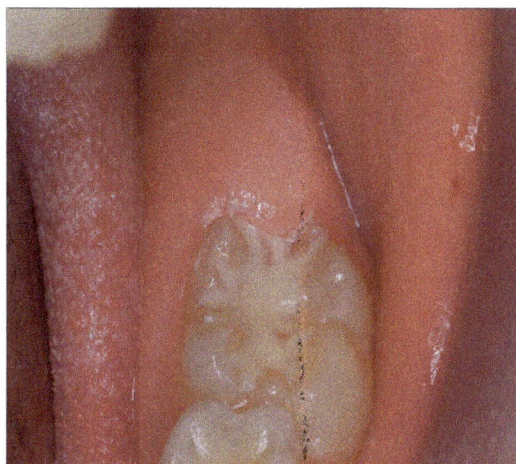

Figure 12. Occlusal view of fissure sealed with nano ionomer cement

7. Retention rates for the fissure sealing

One of the major problems when considering the success rates of sealant restorations is the variation in techniques and materials used. Short term studies indicate a high degree of success for sealant restorations [96-105]. However, longer term studies appear to indicate that success is less predictable [106-110].

Recent study by Gorseta et al. investigated retention of Glass Carbomer fissure sealant after six and twelve months of clinical trial [111]. Glass Carbomer is relatively new material developed from glass ionomer (GIC) and contains nano-sized powder particles and fluorapatite. Advantages of Glass Carbomer comparing to GIC are better mechanical properties and command setting through application of heat. Materials included forty eight teeth with well-delineated fissure morphology divided in two groups which were sealed with Glass Carbomer Sealant (Glass Carbomer Products, Netherlands) and Helioseal F (Vivadent, Liechtenstein) using split mouth design. Investigated materials were placed and set according to manufacturer's instruction using dental light Bluephase 16i (Vivadent, Liechtenstein) (Figure 10). Teeth in group A were sealed with Glass Carbomer material and in group B with Helioseal F. Evaluation criteria (Kilpatrick et al.) for retention of sealant was classified as: type 1: intact sealant; type 2: 1/3 of sealant missing; type 3: 2/3 of sealant missing; and type 4: whole sealant missing. Presence of new caries lesions was evaluated in two categories: 1-absent; 2-present.

Gorseta et al. used replicas for evaluation of fissure sealant retention rate. The impressions with polyvinylxyloxane impression material of Glass Carbomer-sealed teeth were taken in order to obtain replicas of occlusal surfaces (Figure 14). For that purpose, impression was taken and poured in acrylic resin (Citofix Kit, Struers) (Figure 13). The obtained replicas were analysed with SEM (Figure 15, 16).

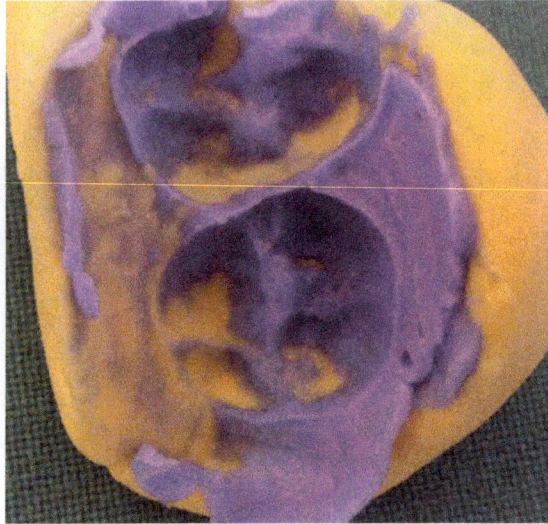

Figure 13. Impression of occlusal surface of molar

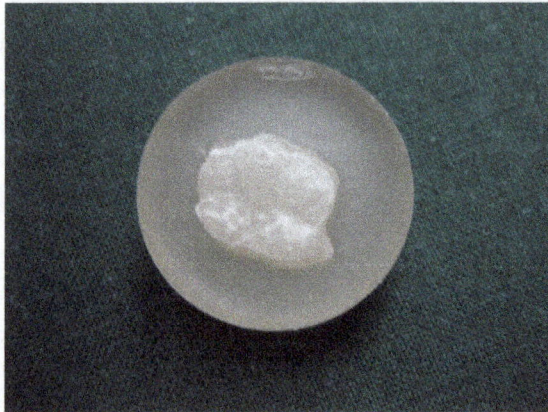

Figure 14. Replicas of occlusal surface of molar

Obtained data were statistically analyzed using non-parametric Mann-Whitney test.

Results showed that retention rate in-group A and B were 100% after six months of clinical service. There were no secondary caries lesions in either group. Results showed that complete retention in group A and B were 75% after 12 months of clinical service. There were two new caries lesions in each group. Mann-Whitney U test doesn't reveal significant statistical difference between groups. Glass Carbomer sealant material showed comparable retention rate to resin based sealant material and can also be recommended for every day practice [111].

In some studies which found statistically significantly more caries in group with glass ionomer sealed teeth at 36-48 months than in group with resin sealed teeth, the complete retention for resin sealants was about 80%, and for glass ionomers was very low (3%) [112, 113, 114].

Studies published by Karlzén-Reuterving and Williams reported similar retention rate did not show a difference between the materials in caries incidence [115, 116]. In next two studies, glass ionomers sealing were reported to be more effective regarding caries prevention [117, 118]. They reported retention of both sealant materials as low (resin-based sealants 28% to 40% and glass ionomers in 21% to 40% after 36 months). Conditioning with 10% polyacrylic acid as well as heating lamp polymerization during curing of cement had no effect on the level of retention of the tested glass ionomer cement (Fuji VII). Similar studies have been done in other parts of Europe, and all with the record of low retention rate of glass ionomer sealants, or the value does not significantly deviate from those of the observed in our study. The two-year Finnish study published the complete retention of polyalcenoic cement at 26% of the sealed teeth compared with 82% fully retained fissure sealants of bis-GMA materials [50].

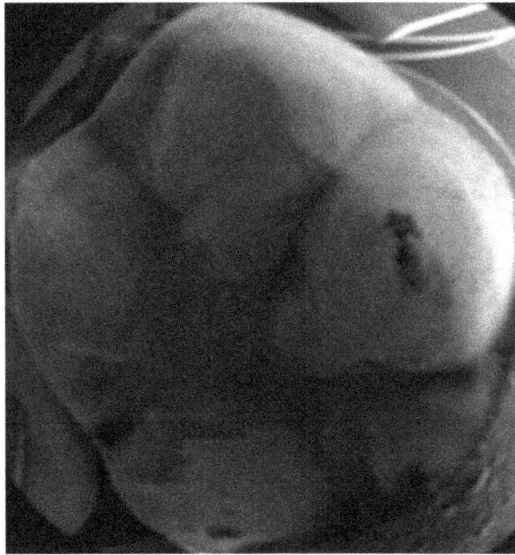

Figure 15. SEM analysis of glass ionomer sealant

After 28 months, Poulsen et al [45] have noted retention of Fuji III of less than 10%, and Pardi et al [46] only 3.5%. After nine months Weerheijm et al. [60] showed an overall retention of Fuji IX in the amount of 51% and only 15% for Fuji III. The incidence of new carious lesions in the group of sealing with glass ionomer cements was not statistically significant. The duration of study is only one year because of the small percentage of retention rate of glass ionomer sealants. Regardless of what is known that the most people prefer chewing on the right side, a control group of sealants (Helioseal F) placed on the right side of the jaw showed a high percentage of retention of 80%.

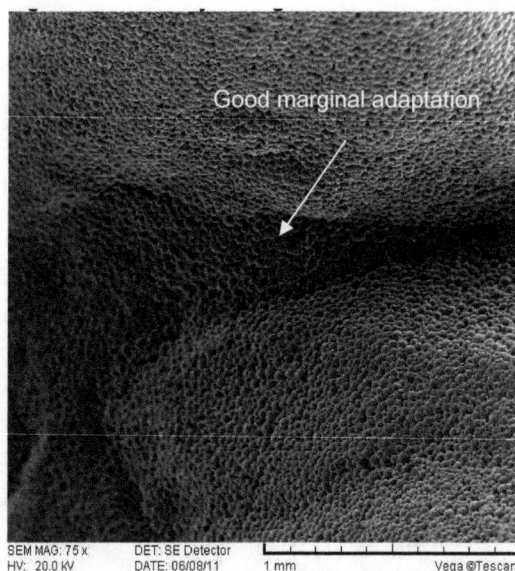

Figure 16. SEM analysis of glass ionomer sealant-higher magnification

Sidhu et al. studied contraction SIC after heating [40]. They concluded that the degree of contraction of the material depends on the porosity within the SIC. These dimensional changes can affect not only the marginal integrity between the enamel and the material, but also compromise the quality of adhesion between the glass ionomer and enamel. As the viscosity of glass ionomers used for sealing fissures greater than the viscosity of the resin sealants, Simonsen, McLean recommend use SIC only fissure having a diameter greater than 100 microns [119]. Also, solutions and gels for fluoridation may affect the surface SIC causing greater roughness [120]. This may induce microfractures on the surface of the material, then the fractures in the material and chained lead to loss of retention of material in the fissure.

The study of Pardi analyzed following sealant materials: flowable resin composite (Revolution), resin-modified glass ionomer (Vitremer) and compomer (DyractFlow) [121]. All occlusal surfaces were conditioned with 37% phosphoric acid. After 2 years, sealants were totally retained on 76% of the teeth sealed with Revolution, on 58% of teeth sealed with Dyract Flow and on 47% of the occlusal surfaces sealed with Vitremer. Recent studies comparing resins to resin-modified glass ionomers at 36 months, reported clearly better complete retention rates for resins (94%) than for resin-modified glass ionomers (5%) [122,123].

There might be many different causes behind the inconsistent results between the studies comparing resin-based materials to glass ionomers as sealants. Therefore, conclusion cannot be drawn based only on retention rate of material as sealants. However, information about caries prevalence in population is very important as diet and oral hygiene [122, 123].

Recent studies showed that the level of retention of glass ionomer sealants treated by heating during setting time is considerably lower than retention of conventional composite resin for sealing. Reduced time manipulation and adhesion of glass ionomer material for the wet surface of the tooth, unequivocally favours glass ionomer material as the material of choice for sealing partially erupted molars [124-130]. This procedure is especially warranted in high caries risk patients, uncooperative patients and those with special needs [121].

Griffin et al. evaluated the effectiveness of sealants in managing caries lesions in a meta-analysis, and found their effectiveness in preventing dentin caries to be in the range of 62% to 100% (median 74% for all; 83% for non-cavitated and 65% for cavitated lesions). They recommended the placement of sealants to arrest lesions in the early carious stages and also to surfaces where caries status is uncertain. The progression of non-cavitated occlusal lesions was slow also for surfaces that were not sealed indicating that such surfaces could either be monitored or sealed. Invasive treatment methods were not recommended [124, 126-131].

Sealant maintenance is an integrated part of the sealant approach – all sealed surfaces should be regularly monitored clinically and radiographically [132-133]. Bitewing radiographs are suggested to be taken at a frequency consistent with the patient's risk status especially in cases where there has been doubt about the surface caries status prior to sealant application [124]. Defective or lost sealants should be reapplied in order to maintain the marginal integrity of sealants.

8. Conclusion

A fissure sealant is a material that is placed in the pits and fissures of teeth in order to prevent or arrest the development of dental caries. As the integrity and retention of a sealant is considered crucial to the success of sealants in the long-term, resin based is the material of choice. Sealing over incipient caries lesions is both effective and practical – the dental profession should be encouraged to use sealants more in an interceptive manner rather than in a preventive or operative manner.) They recommended the placement of sealants to arrest lesions in the early carious stages and also to surfaces where caries status is uncertain. The progression of non-cavitated occlusal lesions was slow also for surfaces that were not sealed indicating that such surfaces could either be monitored or sealed.

Author details

Kristina Goršeta[*]

Address all correspondence to: kgorseta@sfzg.hr

Department of Pediatric and Preventive Dentistry, School of Dental Medicine, University of Zagreb, Croatia

References

[1] Eccles MFW. The problem of occlusal caries and its current management. N Z Dent J. 1989;85(380):50-55.

[2] Bohannan HM. Caries distribution and the case for sealants. J Public Health Dent. 1983; 43(3):200-204.

[3] Ripa LW, Leske GS, Sposato A. The surface-specific caries pattern of participants in a school-based fluoride mouthrinsing program with implications for the use of sealants. J Public Health Dent. 1985;45(2):90-94.

[4] Welbury R., Raadal M., & Lygidakis N.A. EAPD guidelines of the use of pit and fissure sealants. Paediatric Dentistry, 2004.

[5] Nagano T. The form of pits and fissure and the primary lesion of caries. Dent Abstr. 1961;Abstract 6:426.

[6] Slade GD, Spencer AJ, Davies MJ, Burrow D. Intra-oral distribution and impact of caries experience among South Australian School Children. Aust. Dent. J. 1996;41(5): 343–50.

[7] Avinash, J., Marya, C.M., Dhingra, S., Gupta, P., Kataria, S., Meenu, & Bhatia, H. P. Pit and Fissure Sealants: An Unused Caries Prevention Tool. Journal of Oral Health and Community Dentistry, 2010. 4(1), 1-6.

[8] Feigal, R. J., & Donly, K. J. The Use of Pit and Fissure Sealants. Pediatric Dentistry 2006, 28(2), 143-150.5. RE, Haugh LD, Grainger DA Conti AJ. Four-year clinical evaluation of pit and fissure sealant. J Am Dent Assoc. (2006). 1977;95(5):972-981.

[9] Mertz-Fairhurst EJ, Fairhurst CW, Williams JE, Della Giustina VE, Brooks JD. A comparative clinical study of two pit and fissure sealants: 7-year results in Augusta, Georgia. J Am Dent Assoc. 1984;109(2):252-255.

[10] Romcke RG, Lewis DW, Maze BD, Vickerson RA. Retention and maintenance of fissure sealants over 10 years. J Can Dent Assoc. 1990;56(3):235-237.

[11] Donovan, T. E., Anderson, M., Becker, W., Cagna, D. R., Carr, G. B., Albouy, J., Metz, J., Eichmiller, F., & McKee, J. R. Annual Review of selected dental literature: Report of the Committee on Scientific Investigation of the American Academy of Restorative Dentistry. The Journal of Prosthetic Dentistry, (2013). 110(3), 161-210.

[12] Knight, G. M., McIntyre, J. M., Craig, G. G., Zilm, P. S., & Gully, N. J. An in vitro model to measure the effect of a silver fluoride and potassium iodine treatment on the permeability of demineralized dentine to streptococcus mutans Australian Dental Journal, (2005). 50(4), 242-5.

[13] Zero, D. T. How the introduction of the acid-etch technique revolutionized dental practice. The Journal of the American Dental Association, (2013). 144(9), 990-994.

[14] Weintraub JA. The effectivness of pit and fissure sealants. J of Public Health Dent. 1989;49(5 Spec No):317-30.

[15] Welbury R, Raadal M, Lygidakis N. Guidelines on the use of Pit and Fissures Sealants in Paediatric Dentistry. An EAPD policy document. Eur J Paediatr Dent. 2004;3:179-84.

[16] Simonsen RJ. Pit and fissure sealant: review of the literature. Pediatr Dent 2002;24: 393-414.

[17] Adair SM. The role of sealants in caries prevention programs. J Calif Dent Assoc 2003;31:221-7.

[18] Cueto EI, Buonocore MG. Sealing pits and fissures with an adhesive resin. Its use in caries prevention. J Am Dent Assoc. 1967;75(1):121-128.

[19] Gwinnett AJ, Buonocore MG. Adhesives and caries prevention. A preliminary report. Br Dent J. 1965;119:77-80.

[20] Taifour D, Frencken JE, van't Hof MA, Beiruti N, Truin GJ. Effects of glass ionomer sealants in newly erupted first molars after 5 years: a pilot study. Community Dent Oral Epidemiol. 2003;31:314-9.

[21] Poulsen S, Laurberg L, Vaeth M, Jensen U, Haubek D. A field trial of resin-based and glass-ionomer fissure sealants: clinical and radiographic assessment of caries. Community Dent Oral Epidemiol. 2006;34:36-40.

[22] Pardi V, Pereira AC, Mialhe FL, Meneghim MC, Ambrosano GMB. A 5-year evaluation of two glass-ionomer cements used as fissure sealants. Community Dent Oral Epidemiol. 2003;31:386-91.

[23] Forss H, Halme E. Retention of a glass ionomer cement and a resin-based fissure sealant and effect on carious outcome after 7 years. Community Dent Oral Epidemiol. 1998;26:21-5.

[24] Poulsen S, Beiruti N, Sadat N. A comparison of retention and the effect on caries of fissure sealing with a glass-ionomer and a resin-based sealant. Community Dent Oral Epidemiol. 2001;29:298-301.

[25] Williams B, Laxton L, Holt RD, Winter GB. Fissure sealants: a 4-year clinical trial comparing an experimental glass polyalkenoate cement with a bis glycidyl metacrylate resin used as fissure sealants. Br Dent J. 1996;180:104-8.

[26] Mejare I, Major IA. Glass ionomer and resin based fissure sealants: a clinical study. Scand J Dent Res. 1990;98:345-50.

[27] Uribe S. The effectiveness of fissure sealants. Evid Based Dent. 2004;5:92.

[28] Yengopal V, Mickenautsch S, Bezerra A, Leal S. Caries-preventive effect of glass ion-omer and resin-based fissure sealants on permanent teeth: a meta analysis. J Oral Sci 2009;51(3):373–82.

[29] Seth, S. (2011). Glass ionomer cement and resin-based fissure sealants are equally effective in caries prevention. JADA, 142(5), 551-552.

[30] Ahovuo-Saloranta, A., Forss, H., Walsh, T., Hiiri, A., Nordblad, A., Mäkelä, M., & Worthington, H. V. (2012). Sealants for preventing dental decay in the permanent teeth. The Cochrane database of systematic reviews, 3, 1-139.

[31] Ahovuo-Saloranta A, Hiiri A, Nordblad A, Mäkelä M, Worthington HV. Pit and fissure sealants for preventing dental decay in the permanent teeth of children and adolescents. Cochrane Database of Systematic Reviews 2008, Issue 4. [DOI: 10.1002/14651858.CD001830.pub3]

[32] Mejare I, Lingstrom P, Petersson L, Holm AK, Twetman S, Kallestal C, et al. Caries preventive effect of fissure sealants: a systematic review. Acta Odontol Scand 2003;61(6):321–30.

[33] Feigal RJ. The use of pit and fissure sealants. Pediatr Dent 2002; 24: 415-22.

[34] Feigal RJ. Sealants and preventive restorations: review of effectiveness and clinical changes for improvement. Pediatric Dent.1998;20(2):85-92.

[35] Seleeman JB, Owens BM, Johnson WW. Effect of preparation technique, fissure morphology, and material characteristics on the in vitro margin permeability and penetrability of pit and fissure sealants. Pediatr Dent. 2007; 29(4):308-314.

[36] Llodra JC, Bravo M, Delgado-Rodriguez M, Baca P, Galvez R. Factors influencing the effectiveness of sealants-a metaanalysis. Community Dentistry and Oral Epidemiology 1993; 21(5):261–8.

[37] Splieth CH, Ekstrand KR, Alkilzy M, Clarkson J, MeyerLueckel H, Martignon S, et. al. Sealants in dentistry: outcomes of the ORCA Saturday Afternoon Symposium 2007. Caries Research 2010;44(1):3–13.

[38] McLean JW, Wilson AD. Fissure sealing and filling with an adhesive glass-ionomer cement. British Dental Journal 1974;136(7):269–76.

[39] Algera TJ, Kleverlaan CJ, de Gee AJ, Prahl-Andersen B, Feilzer AJ. The influence of accelerating the setting rate by ultrasound or heat on the bond strength of glass ionomers used as ortodontic bracket cements. Eur J Orthod. 2005;27:472-6.

[40] Sidhu SK, Carrick TE, McCabe JF. Temperature mediated coefficient of dimensional change of dental tooth-colored restorative materials. Dent Mater 2004;20: 435–440.

[41] Skrinjaric K, Vranic DN, Glavina D, Skrinjaric I. Heat treated glass ionomer cement fissure sealants: retention after 1 year follow-up. International Journal of Paediatric-Dentistry 2008;18(5):368–73.

[42] Morphis TL, Toumba KJ. Retention of two fluoride pit-and-fissure sealants in comparison to a conventional sealant. Int J Paediatr Dent. 1998;8:203-8.

[43] Walker J, Floyd K, Jakobsen J. The effectiveness of sealants in pediatric patients. J Dent Child. 1996;63:268-70.

[44] Lygidakis NA, Oulis KI, Christodoulidis A. Evaluation of fissure sealants retention following four different isolation and surface preparation techniques: four years clinical trial. J Clin Pediatr Dent. 1994;19:23-5.

[45] Poulsen S, Laurberg L, Vaeth M, Jensen U, Haubek D. A field trial of resin-based and glass-ionomer fissure sealants: clinical and radiographic assessment of caries. Community Dent Oral Epidemiol. 2006;34:36-40.

[46] Pardi V, Pereira AC, Mialhe FL, Meneghim MC, Ambrosano GMB. A 5-year evaluation of two glass-ionomer cements used as fissure sealants. Community Dent Oral Epidemiol. 2003;31:386-91.

[47] Forss H, Halme E. Retention of a glass ionomer cement and a resin-based fissure sealant and effect on carious outcome after 7 years. Community Dent Oral Epidemiol. 1998;26:21-5.

[48] Poulsen S, Beiruti N, Sadat N. A comparison of retention and the effect on caries of fissure sealing with a glass-ionomer and a resin-based sealant. Community Dent Oral Epidemiol. 2001;29:298-301.

[49] Williams B, Laxton L, Holt RD, Winter GB. Fissure sealants: a 4-year clinical trial comparing an experimental glass polyalkenoate cement with a bis glycidyl metacrylate resin used as fissure sealants. Br Dent J. 1996;180:104-8.

[50] Forss H, Saarni M, Seppa L. Comparison of glass ionomer and resin based sealants. Community Dent Oral Epidemiol. 1994;22:21-4.

[51] Dennison JB, Straffon LH, More FG. Evaluating tooth eruption on sealant efficacy. J Am Dent Assoc 1990 Nov;121(5):610-4.

[52] Walker J, Floyd K, Jakobsen J, Pinkham JR. The effectiveness of preventive resin restorations in pediatric patients. ASDC J Dent Child 1996 Sep-Oct;63(5):338-40.

[53] Cueto EI, Buonocore MG. Sealing of pits and fissures with an adhesive resin: its use in caries prevention. J Am Dent Assoc 1967Jul;75(1):121-8.

[54] Chestnutt IG, Schafer F, Jacobson AP, Stephen KW. The prevalence and effectiveness of fissure sealants in Scottish adolescents. Br Dent J 1994 Aug 20;177(4):125-9.

[55] Jo E. Frencken. The ART approach using glass-ionomers in relation to global oral health care. Dental materials 2010;26:1–6.)

[56] Simonsen RJ. Retention and effectiveness of a single application of white sealant after 10 years. J Am Dent Assoc. 1987115(1):31-36.

[57] Simonsen RJ. Retention and effectiveness of dental sealant after 15 years. J Am Dent Assoc. 1991;122(10):34-42.

[58] Goršeta, Kristina; Škrinjarić, Tomislav; Glavina, Domagoj. The effect of heating and ultrasound on the shear bond strength of glass ionomer cement. // Collegium antropologicum. 36 (2012), 4; 1307-1312

[59] Uribe S. The effectiveness of fissure sealants. Evid Based Dent. 2004;5:92.

[60] Weerheijm KL, Kreulen CM, Gruythuysen RJM. Comparison of retentive qualities of two glass-ionomer cements used as fissure sealants. J Dent Child. 1996;63:265-7.

[61] Taifour D, Frencken JE, van't Hof MA, Beiruti N, Truin GJ. Effects of glass ionomer sealants in newly erupted first molars after 5 years: a pilot study. Community Dent Oral Epidemiol. 2003;31:314-9.

[62] Mejare I, Major IA. Glass ionomer and resin based fissure sealants: a clinical study. Scand J Dent Res. 1990;98:345-50.

[63] Ahovuo-Saloranta A, Hiri A, Nordblad A, Worthington H, Mäkelä M. Pit and fissure sealants for preventing dental decay in the permanent teeth of children and adolescents. Cohrane Database Syst Rev [serial on the internet]. 2004 [cited 2007 Apr 16]; Issue 3: CD001830.pub.2. DOI: 10.1002/14651858.CD00183.pub2. Available from: www.ncbi.nlm.mih.gov

[64] Hill RG, Wilson AD. Some structural aspects of glasses used in glass ionomer cements. Glass Technol. 1988;29:150-88.

[65] Pereira AC, Eggertsson H, Martinez-Mier EA, Mialhe FL, Eckert GJ, Zero DT. Validity of caries detection on occlusal surfaces and treatment decisions based on results from multiple caries-detection methods. Eur J Oral Sci 2009;117(1):51–7.

[66] Tranaeus S, Shi XQ, Angmar-Mansson B. Caries risk assessment: methods available to clinicians for caries detection. Community Dent Oral Epidemiol 2005;33(4):265–73.

[67] Zandona AF and Zero DT. Diagnostic tools for early caries detection. J Am Dent Assoc 2006;137(12):1675–84.

[68] Baelum V, Heidmann J, Nyvad B. Dental caries paradigms in diagnosis and diagnostic research. Eur J Oral Sci 2006;114(4):263–77.

[69] Beiruti N, Frencken JE, van't Hof MA, Taifour D, van Palenstein Helderman WH. Caries-preventive effect of a one-time application of composite resin and glass ionome-sealants after 5 years Caries Research 2006;40(1):52–9.

[70] McComb D, Tam LE. Diagnosis of occlusal caries: Part I. Conventional methods. Journal of Canadian Dental Association 2001;67(8):454–7.

[71]   Bader JD, Shugars DA. A systematic review of the performance of a laser fluores-
       cence device for detecting caries. Journal of the American Dental Association
       2004;135 (10):1413–26.

[72]   Lussi A, Hibst R, Paulus R. DIAGNOdent: an optical method for caries detection.
       Journal of Dental Research 2004;83(Spec Iss C):C80–3.

[73]   Beauchamp J. CPW, Crall J.J., Donly K., Feigal R., Gooch B., Ismail A., Kohn W., Sie-
       gal M., Simonsen R. Evidence-based clinical recommendations for the use of pit-and-
       fissure sealants: A report of the American Dental Association Council on Scientific
       Affairs. JADA. 2008; 139

[74]   Ekstrand KR, Martignon S, Ricketts DJN, Qvist V. Detection and activity assessment
       of primary coronal caries lesions: a methodologic study. Oper Dent 2007;32(3):225–
       35.

[75]   Bader JD, Shugars DA, Bonito AJ. A systematic review of the performance of meth-
       ods for identifying carious lesions. J Public Health Dent 2002;62(4):201–13.

[76]   Ismail AI, Sohn W, Tellez M, Amaya A, Sen A, Hasson H, et al. The International Ca-
       ries Detection and Assessment System (ICDAS): an integrated system for measuring
       dental caries. Community Dent Oral Epidemiol 2007;35(3):170–8.

[77]   Raadal M, Espelid I, Mejare I. The caries lesion and its management in children and
       adolescents. In: Pediatric Dentistry: a clinical approach. Koch G, Poulsen S (eds). Co-
       penhagen: Munksgaard; 2001. pp. 173-212.

[78]   Harris NO, Garcia-Godoy F. Primary preventive dentistry. 5th edition. London: Asi-
       mon and Schuster Company; 1999.

[79]   Goldstein RE, Parkins FM. Air-abrasive technology: its new role in restorative den-
       tistry. JADA 1994;125:551-7.

[80]   De Craene GP, Martens C, Dermaut R. The invasive pit and fissure sealing technique
       in pediatric dentistry: an SEM study of a preventive restoration. ASDC J Dent Child
       1988;55(1):34-42.

[81]   Waggoner WF, Siegal M. Pit and fissure sealant application: updating the technique.
       J Am Dent Assoc 1996 Mar;127(3):351-61, quiz 391-2.

[82]   Shapira J, Eidelman E. Six-year clinical evaluation of fissure sealants placed after me-
       chanical preparation: a matched pair study. Pediatr Dent 1986 Sep;8(3):204-5.

[83]   Lygidakis NA, Oulis KI, Christodoulidis A. Evaluation of fissure sealants retention
       following four different isolation and surface preparation techniques: four years clin-
       ical trial. J Clin Pediatr Dent 1994 Fall;19(1):23-5.

[84]   Blackwood JA, Dilley DC, Roberts MW, Swift EJ Jr. Evaluation of pumice, fissure en-
       ameloplasty and air abrasion on sealant microleakage. Pediatr Dent 2002 May-Jun;
       24(3):199-203.

[85]   Christensen GJ. Fluoride made it: why haven't sealants? JADA 1992;123(2):89-90.

[86]   Donnan MF, Ball IA. A double-blind clinical trial to determine the importance of pumice prophylaxis on fissure sealant retention. Br Dent J 1988 Oct 22;165(8):283-6.

[87]   Silverstone LM. State of the art on sealant research and priorities for further research. J Dent Educ 1984 Feb;48 (2 Suppl):10718.

[88]   Cooper TM. Four-handed dentistry in the team practice of dentistry. Dent Clin North Am 1974;18(4):739-753.

[89]   Robinson GE, Wuehrmann AH, Sinnett GM, McDevitt EJ. Fourhanded dentistry: the whys and wherefores. JADA 1968; 77(3):573-579.

[90]   Wood AJ, Saravia ME, Farrington FH. Cotton roll isolation versus Vac-Ejector isolation. ASDC J Dent Child 1989;56:438-41.

[91]   Manton DJ, Messer LB. Pit and fissure sealants: another major cornerstone in preventive dentistry. Aust Dent J 1995 Feb;40(1):22-9.

[92]   Duggal MS, Tahmassebi JF, Toumba KJ, Mavromati C. The effect of different etching times on the retention of fissure sealants in second primary and first permanent molars. Int J Paediatr Dent 1997 Jun;7(2):81-6.

[93]   Barroso JM, Lessa FC, Palma Dibb RG, Torres CP, Pecora J, Borsatto MC. Shear bond strength of pit and fissure sealants to saliva contaminated and non-contaminated enamel. J Dent Child 2005;72:95-9.

[94]   Chosak A, Eidelman E. Effect of time from application until exposure to light on the tag lengths of a visible light-polymerized sealant. Dent Mater 1988;4:302-6.

[95]   Dennison JB, Straffon LH, More FG.Evaluating tooth eruption on sealant efficacy. JADA 1990;121:610-4.

[96]   Simonsen RJ, Stallard RE. Sealantrestorations utilizing a dilute filled composite resin: one year results. Quintessence Int 1977;23:307-315.

[97]   Azhdari S, Sveen OB, Buonocore MG. Evaluation of a restorative preventive technique for localized occlusal caries. J Dent Res 1979;58(special issue A):330 Abstract 952.

[98]   Walker JD, Jensen ME, Pickham JR. A clinical review of preventive resin restorations. ASDC J Dent Child 1990;57:257-259.

[99]   Houpt M, Eidelman E, Shey Z, et al. Occlusal restoration using fissure sealant instead of 'extension for prevention', eighteen month results. J Dent Res 1982;61:214. Abstract 324.

[100] Gray G B. An evaluation of sealant restorations after 2 years. Br Dent J 1999;186:569-575.

[101] Walls AWG, Murray JJ, McCabe JF. The management of occlusal caries in permanent molars. A clinical trial comparing a minimal composite restoration with an occlusal amalgam restoration. Br Dent J 1988;164:288-292.

[102] Simonsen RJ, Jensen ME. Preventive resin restorations utilizing a diluted filled composite resins: 30 months results. J Dent Res 1979;58(special issue A):330(abstract No. 952).

[103] Raadal M. Follow-up study of sealing and filling with composite resins in the prevention of occlusal caries. Community Dent Oral Epidemiol 1978;6:176-180.

[104] Simonsen RJ. Preventive resin restorations. J Am Dent Assoc 1980;100:535-539.

[105] Houpt M, Eidelman E, Shey EZ. Occlusal restoration using fissure sealant instead of 'extension for prevention'. ASCD J Dent Child 1984;51:270-273.

[106] Houpt M, Eidelman E, Shey EZ. Occlusal composite restorations:4 year results. J Am Dent Assoc 1985;110:351-353.

[107] Welbury RR, Walls AGW, Murray JJ, McCabe JF. The management of occlusal caries in permanent molars. A 5-year clinical trial comparing a minimal composite with an amalgam restoration. Br Dent J 1990;169:361-366.

[108] Houpt M, Fuks A, Eidelman E. Composite/sealant restoration: 6.5 year results. Paed Dent 1988; 10: 304-306.

[109] Simonsen RJ, Landy NA. Preventive Resin Restorations: fracture resistance and 7-year clinical results. J Dent Res 1984; 63(special issue): 261(abstract No.175).

[110] Houpt M, Fuks A, Eidelman E. The preventive resin (composite resin/sealant) restoration:Nine-year results. Quintessence Int 1994;25:155-159.

[111] K. Gorseta, D. Glavina, A. Borzabadi-Farahani, R.N. Van Duinen, I. Skrinjaric, R.G. Hill and E. Lynch. One-Year Clinical Evaluation of a Glass Carbomer Fissure Sealant, a Preliminary Study European Journal of Prosthodontics and Restorative Dentistry. 22 (2014), 2; 67-71.

[112] Kervanto-Seppälä S, Lavonius E, Pietilä I, Pitkäniemi J, Meurman J, Kerosuo E. Comparing the caries-preventive effect of two fissure sealing modalities in public health care: a single application of glass ionomer and a routine resin-based sealant programme. A randomized split-mouth clinical trial. International Journal of Paediatric Dentistry 2008;18(1):56–61.

[113] Poulsen S, Beiruti N, Sadat N. A comparison of retention and the effect on caries of fissure sealing with a glassionomer and a resin-based sealant. Community Dentistry and Oral Epidemiology 2001;29(4):298–301.

[114] Rock WP, Foulkes EE, Perry H, Smith AJ. A comparative study of fluoride-releasing composite resin and glass ionomer materials used as fissure sealants. Journal of Dentistry 1996;24(4):275–80.

[115] Karlzén-Reuterving G, van Dijken JW. A three-year followup of glass ionomer cement and resin fissure sealants. Journal of Dentistry for Children 1995;62(2):108–10.

[116] Williams B, Laxton L, Holt RD, Winter GB. Fissure sealants: a 4-year clinical trial comparing an experimental glass polyalkenoate cement with a bis glycidyl methacrylate resin used as fissure sealants. British Dental Journal 1996; 180(3):104–8.

[117] Arrow P, Riordan PJ. Retention and caries preventive effects of a GIC and a resin-based fissure sealant. Community Dentistry and Oral Epidemiology 1995;23(5):282–5.

[118] Beiruti N, Frencken JE, van't Hof MA, Taifour D, van Palenstein Helderman WH. Caries-preventive effect of a one-time application of composite resin and glass ionome-sealants after 5 years. Caries Research 2006;40(1):52–9.

[119] McLean JW, Wilson AD. Fissure sealing and filling with an adhesive glass-ionomer cement. Br Dent J. 1974;136:269-76.

[120] De Witte AM, De Maeyer EA, Verbeeck RM. Surface roughening of glass ionomer cements by neutral NaF solutions. Biomater. 2003;24:1995-2000.

[121] Pardi V, Pereira AC, Ambrosano GMB, Meneghim MdeC. Clinical evaluation of three different materials used as pit and fissure sealant: 24-months results. Journal of Clinical Pediatric Dentistry 2005;29(2):133–8.

[122] Baseggio W, Naufel FS, Davidoff DC, Nahsan FP, Flury S, Rodrigues JA. Caries-preventive efficacy and retention of a resin-modified glass ionomer cement and a resin-based fissure sealant: a 3-year split-mouth randomised clinical trial. Oral Health & Preventive Dentistry 2010;8(3):261–8.

[123] Raadal M, Utkilen AB, Nilsen OL. Fissure sealing with light-cured resin-reinforced glass-ionomer cement (Vitrebond) compared with a resin sealant. International Journal of Paediatric Dentistry 1996;6(4):235–9.

[124] Griffin SO, Oong E, Kohn W, Vidakovic B, Gooch BF, CDC Dental Sealant Systematic Review Work Group, et al. The effectiveness of sealants in managing caries lesions. J Dent Res (2008). 87(2):169-74.

[125] Chen X, Du M, Fan M, Mulder J, Huysmans MC, Frencken JE. Effectiveness of two new types of sealants: retention after 2 years. Clinical Oral Investigations 2012;16(5): 1443–50.

[126] Barja-Fidalgo F, Maroun S, de Oliveira BH. Effectiveness of a glass ionomer cement used as a pit and fissure sealant in recently erupted permanent first molars. Journal of Dentistry for Children 2009;76(1):34–40.

[127] Liu BY, Lo ECM, Chu CH, Lin HC. Randomized trial on fluorides and sealants for fissure caries prevention. Journal of Dental Research 2012;91(8):753–8.

[128] Beiruti N, Frencken JE, van't Hof MA, Taifour D, van Palenstein Helderman WH. Caries-preventive effect of one-time application of composite resin and glass ionome-sealants after 5 years. Caries Research 2006;40(1):52–9.

[129] Antonson SA, Antonson DE, Brener S, Crutchfield J, Larumbe J, Michaud C, et al.Twenty-four month clinical evaluation of fissure sealants on partially erupted permanent first molars: glass ionomer versus resin-based sealant. Journal of the American Dental Association 2012;143(2): 115–22.

[130] Yilmaz Y, Beldüz N, Eyübo lu O. A two-year evaluation of four different fissure sealants. European Archives of Paediatric Dentistry: Official Journal of the European Academy of Paediatric Dentistry 2010;11(2):88–92.

[131] Yildiz E, Dörter C, Efes B, Koray F. A comparative study of two fissure sealants: a 2-year clinical follow-up. Journal of Oral Rehabilitation 2004;31(10):979–84.

[132] Yakut N, Sönmez H. Resin composite sealant vs. polyacidmodified resin composite applied to post eruptive mature and immature molars: two year clinical study. The Journal of Clinical Pediatric Dentistry 2006;30(3):215–8.

[133] Taifour D, Frencken JE, van't Hof MA, Beiruti N, Truin GJ. Effects of a glass ionomer sealant in newly erupted first molars after 5 years: a pilot study. Community Dentistry and Oral Epidemiology 2003;31(4):314–9.

8

Oral Health and Adverse Pregnancy Outcomes

Sukumaran Anil, Raed M. Alrowis,
Elna P. Chalisserry, Vemina P. Chalissery,
Hani S. AlMoharib and Asala F. Al-Sulaimani

1. Introduction

Maternal health has long been recognized as an important determinant in reducing the risk for pregnancy-related complications such as preterm birth and preeclampsia. Preterm (PTB) delivery and low birth weight (LBW) are considered to be the most relevant biological determinants of newborn infant survival in both developed and developing countries. The oral changes that can occur in pregnancy have been a focus of interest for many years. Physiological changes that occur in pregnant women can adversely affect oral health. Elevations in estrogen and progesterone enhance the inflammatory response and consequently alter the gingival tissue (Mascarenhas et al., 2003). During pregnancy, the incidences of gingivitis and periodontitis are increased, and many pregnant women suffer from bleeding and spongy gums.

Periodontal disease, a persistent bacterial infection, leads to a chronic and systemic challenge with bacterial substances and host-derived inflammatory mediators that are capable of initiating and promoting systemic diseases (Williams et al., 2000; Gibbs, 2001). The mechanisms underlying this destructive process involve both direct tissue damage resulting from bacterial products and indirect damage through bacterial induction of the host inflammatory and immune responses. Even though controversy exists regarding the role of oral health as an independent contributor to abnormal pregnancy outcomes, the recognition and understanding of the importance of oral health has led to significant research into the role of maternal oral health in pregnancy outcomes (Sanz et al., 2013). Adequate oral hygiene habits are mandatory to control the development of periopathogenic oral biofilms, which have been reported to be associated with poor obstetric outcomes (Lieff et al., 2004; Han, 2011).

The chapter will cover the following aspects on oral health and adverse pregnancy outcomes including a systematic analysis of the studies linking preterm delivery, low birth weight, preeclampsia and periodontal disease.

- Association between periodontitis and pregnancy.
- Pre term birth, low birth weight and periodontal disease.
- Preeclampsia and periodontal disease.
- Biological mechanism linking periodontal disease to adverse pregnancy outcome.
- Evidence based literature analysis.
- Observational and systematic studies.
- Intervention studies on the impact of periodontal therapy
- Other expected oral outcomes due to pregnancy
- Early childhood caries.
- Gingival enlargement.

2. Association between periodontitis and pregnancy

Several studies have revealed the role and influence of periodontitis on adverse pregnancy outcomes. During pregnancy, the changes in hormone levels promote an inflammatory response that increases the risk of developing gingivitis and periodontitis. Even with good plaque control, 50%-70% of all women will develop gingivitis during their pregnancy, commonly referred to as pregnancy gingivitis, due to the variations in hormone levels. Pregnancy gingivitis generally manifests during the second and eighth months of pregnancy and is considered a consequence of the observed increased levels of the hormones progesterone and estrogen, which can effect small blood vessels of the gingiva, making it more permeable (Jensen et al., 1981; Barak et al., 2003).

Research suggests that the presence of maternal periodontitis has been associated with adverse pregnancy outcomes such as preterm birth (Offenbacher et al., 1996; Jeffcoat et al., 2001; Offenbacher et al., 2001), preeclampsia (Boggess et al., 2003), gestational diabetes (Xiong et al., 2006), delivery of a small-for-gestational-age infant, and fetal loss (Moore et al., 2004; Boggess et al., 2006). These increased risks suggest that periodontitis may be an independent risk factor for adverse pregnancy outcomes.

3. Preterm, Low Birth Weight (LBW) and periodontal disease

Preterm (PTB) delivery is defined as delivery before 37 weeks of gestation. The international definition of low birth weight (LBW), adopted by the 29th World Health assembly in 1976, is a birth weight of less than 2,500 grams (WHO, 1984). The primary cause of LBW is PTB delivery or premature rupture of membranes. Preterm infants who are born with a low birth weight are termed preterm low birth weight (PLBW). PTB and LBW are considered to be the most relevant biological determinants of newborn infants survival, both in developed and in developing countries. Preterm birth is a major cause of infant mortality and morbidity and poses considerable medical and economic burdens on society (Alves and Ribeiro, 2006). The rate of preterm birth appears to be increasing worldwide, and efforts to prevent or reduce its prevalence have been largely unsuccessful. The importance of PTB and LBW deliveries comes from their capacity to predict the increased risk of mortality among infants born with this condition. Preterm births account for 75% of perinatal mortality and more than half of long-term morbidity (Goldenberg et al., 2008). Moreover, one of the targets of the World Health Organization is to reduce the number of births in which the child weighs less than 2,500 g because this is a known predictor of childhood morbidity and mortality (Cruz et al., 2005).

The primary factors causing LBW infant deliveries are high or low maternal age (>34 yrs or <17 yrs.), smoking, alcohol or drug use during pregnancy, inadequate prenatal care, race, maternal demographic characteristics, hypertension, psychological characteristics, adverse behaviors, multiple pregnancies, nutritional status, diabetes, genitourinary tract infections, uterine contractions and cervical length, and biological and genetic markers (Verkerk et al., 1993; Copper et al., 1996; Nordstrom and Cnattingius, 1996; Romero et al., 2002; Marakoglu et al., 2008).

Microbiological studies suggest that intrauterine infection might account for 25–40% of preterm births. Microorganisms can gain access to the amniotic cavity by (1) ascending from the vagina and the cervix; (2) hematogenous dissemination through the placenta; (3) accidental introduction during invasive procedures; and (4) retrograde spreading through the fallopian tubes (Goldenberg et al., 2000). It has been suggested that spontaneous preterm labor is commonly associated with bacterial vaginosis, a vaginal condition characterized by the prevalence of anaerobes (Gibbs, 2001). This has been shown to elicit an inflammatory burden that results in placental damage and distress and, hence, fetal growth restriction. In addition, the cascade of disordered cytokine response can lead to the stimulation of prostaglandin synthesis and the release of matrix metalloproteinases (MMPs), which account for the uterine contractions and membrane rupture, respectively, and lead to the induction of labor (Romero et al., 1992; Winkler et al., 1998). This suggests that distant sites of infection (oral cavity) or sepsis may target the placental membranes. The maternal susceptibility to oral infections during pregnancy increases the sensitivity of the gingiva to the pathogenic bacteria found in dental biofilms (Barak et al., 2003). Studies have reported the presence of higher levels of *Porphyromonas gingivalis, Bacteroides forsythus, Actinobacillus actinomycetemcomitans* and *Treponema denticola*, organisms normally associated with periodontal disease, in mothers of PTB and LBW babies as compared to normal controls (Offenbacher et al., 1996). Approximately 25% of PLBW deliveries occur without any of the risk factors discussed in this section, which emphasizes the limited understanding of the causes and pathophysiology of the problem (McGaw, 2002).

In 1996, researchers first reported a relationship between maternal periodontal disease and the delivery of a preterm infant. The 1996 study by Offenbacher and colleagues suggested that maternal periodontal disease could lead to a seven-fold increased risk of delivering a PLBW infant. Since then, researchers have investigated these possible associations for over a decade. It is important to understand the underlying biologic mechanisms for the relationship between periodontal disease and adverse pregnancy outcomes such as preterm birth to provide a rationale for therapeutic interventions and exploration of other methods that may be used as adjuncts to the standard treatment. These authors concluded that approximately 18% of PLBW cases might be attributable to periodontal disease (Offenbacher et al., 1996).

4. Preeclampsia and periodontal disease

Preeclampsia is a complication recognized by gestational hypertension and proteinuria. It is one of the most significant health problems during pregnancy and affects 8% to 10% of all pregnancies (Roberts et al., 2003). Intravascular inflammation and endothelial cell dysfunction with altered placental vascular development is believed to be central to the pathogenesis of preeclampsia. To prevent fetal morbidity due to preeclampsia, preterm delivery is induced (Boggess et al., 2006). Maternal clinical periodontal disease at delivery has been associated with an increased risk for the development of preeclampsia (Canakci et al., 2007).

Boggess et al. (2003) were the first investigators to report an association between maternal clinical periodontal infection and the development of preeclampsia. In this longitudinal study, they found a two-fold increased risk for preeclampsia among women with periodontal disease during pregnancy compared with controls. A few other studies also reported an association between preeclampsia and periodontal disease (Table). Canakci et al. (2007) reported that women with preeclampsia were three times more likely to have periodontal infections than healthy women and that periodontal disease also affects the severity of preeclampsia. Barak and colleagues (2007) also found that women with preeclampsia experienced more severe periodontitis than healthy controls. They found a significant elevation in the gingival crevicular fluid levels of PGE-2, interleukin (IL)-1 P, and tumor necrosis factor alpha (TNF-a). In their study, Contreras et al. (2006) found more severe periodontal infections in pregnant women with preeclampsia with the presence of *P. gingivalis, T. forsythensis,* and *E. corrodens* than in controls.

5. Biological mechanism linking periodontal disease to adverse pregnancy outcomes

Two potential mechanisms have been put forward to explain the underlying link between oral health and adverse pregnancy outcomes (Han, 2011). First, periodontal disease causes systemic abnormal immunological changes, leading to pregnancy complications. The elevated systemic inflammation leads to elevated C-reactive protein (CRP) levels, which increase the risk for preeclampsia. Translocation of oral bacteria into the placenta has been demonstrated in animal models of both chronic and acute infections (Lin et al., 2003b; Han et al., 2004).

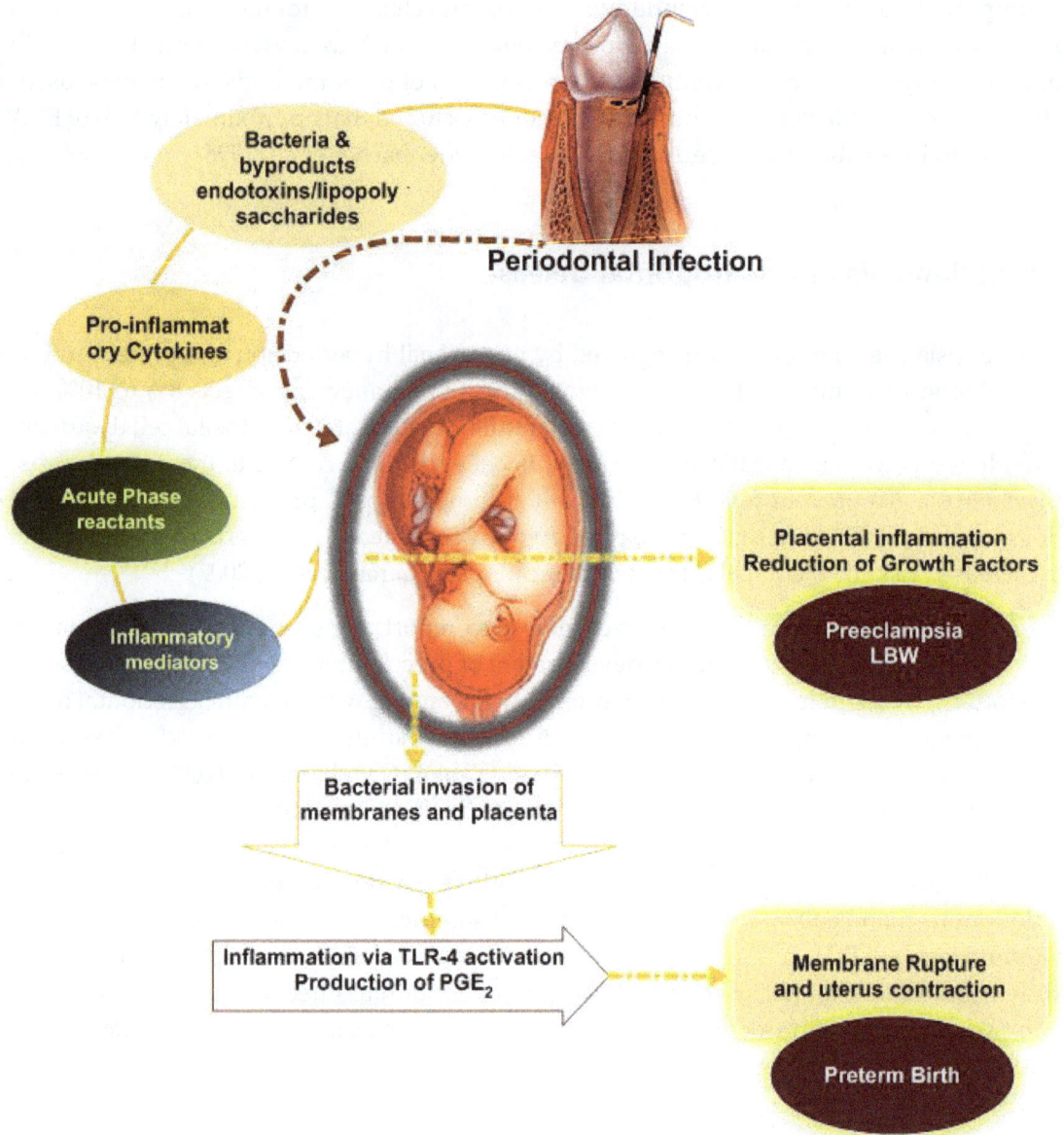

Figure 1. Possible biological mechanism linking periodontal disease and pregnancy complications.

The biological mechanisms proposed to explain the link between maternal periodontitis and PLBW involve the translocation of either inflammatory mediators such as IL-1 β, TNFα and PGE$_2$ or periodontal bacteria and their products from the periodontal tissues to the fetal-placental unit via the systemic circulation, thereby triggering preterm labor (Hillier et al., 1988). Increased levels of interleukin-1 beta (IL-1β), IL-6, tumor necrosis factor alpha (TNF-α, beta-glucuronidase (β–glucuronidase), prostaglandin E2 (PGE2), aspartate aminotransferase (AST), and metalloproteinase-8 (MMPT-8) and decreased levels of osteoprotegerin (OPG) have been detected not only in the gingival tissues, gingival crevicular fluid (GCF), and saliva but also in the serum/plasma of patients affected by periodontal disease (Lin et al., 2003a; Offenbacher et al., 2006; Furugen et al., 2008; Trindade et al., 2008; Wright et al., 2008; Duarte et al., 2010; Buduneli and Kinane, 2011).

Cytokines such as IL-1, IL-6, and TNF-α are all potent inducers of both prostaglandin synthesis and labor, and the levels of these cytokines have been found to be elevated in the amniotic fluid of patients with amniotic fluid infections in preterm labor (Romero et al., 2006). The intra-amniotic levels of PGE_2 and TNF-α rise steadily throughout pregnancy until a critical threshold is reached to induce labor, cervical dilation, and delivery (Offenbacher et al., 1996). Lipo poly sacchrides (LPS), one of the microbial components, can activate macrophages and other cells to synthesize and secrete a wide array of molecules, including the cytokines IL-16, TNF-α, and IL-6, PGE2 and matrix metalloproteinases (Darveau et al., 1997).

The second hypothesis suggests that oral bacteria directly colonize the placenta, causing a localized inflammatory response that results in prematurity and other adverse outcomes. The ratio of anaerobic gram-negative bacterial species to aerobic species increases in dental plaques during the second trimester of pregnancy (Kornman and Loesche, 1980), which may lead to increased cytokine production. If these bacteria escape into the general circulation and cross the placental barrier, they could augment the physiologic levels of PGE_2 and TNF-α in the amniotic fluid and induce premature labor. Animal studies have shown that chronic maternal exposure to the periodontal pathogen *P. gingivalis* results in systemic dissemination, transpla-cental passage, and fetal exposure (Lin et al., 2003b; Boggess et al., 2005). Studies in murine models have shown that *P. gingivalis* infection compromises normal fetal development by systemic dissemination and direct targeting of the fetal-placental unit.

6. Observational studies

The increasing number of case control studies investigating a link between periodontal disease and various adverse pregnancy outcomes in humans has produced conflicting findings (Table 1, 2, 3). Several studies suggest a significant association between maternal periodontal disease and pregnancy complications, including premature delivery, low birth weight and preeclamp-sia. Periodontal disease and progression during pregnancy appear to confer risk for preterm delivery, and the strength of the association increases at earlier gestational deliveries. However, not all studies supported this contention. Differences in the ethnicity and levels of periodontal disease in patients have been proposed as possible reasons for the conflicting findings reported in these studies. Periodontal disease is twice as prevalent among African-Americans, and this might possibly explain the observed increased risk in preterm delivery and fetal growth restriction among African-Americans (Madianos et al., 2001).Adverse pregnancy outcome and periodontal disease share a number of common risk factors, including age, ethnicity, socioeconomic status and smoking. The majority of studies investigating this association have used a dichotomous definition based on the number of teeth or sites with predefined levels of probing depth and attachment loss. Other studies have employed a range of continuous variables to reflect periodontal status, including probing depth, attachment loss and bleeding on probing. Several studies focused on the clinical measures of periodontal disease, which may not adequately reflect the infectious/ inflammatory burden present in pregnant women. The effect of periodontal disease on adverse pregnancy outcome suggests that periodontal infection as a risk factor but the evidence is insufficient to establish a cause and effect relationship.

7. Interventional studies

Several studies have examined the effects of periodontal treatment on preterm birth and low birth weight outcomes with conflicting findings (Table.4). Studies showed that periodontal therapy provided to women with periodontitis or gingivitis during pregnancy reduced the incidence of preterm low birth weight compared to those whose treatment was delayed until after birth (Lopez et al., 2002; Jeffcoat et al., 2003; Lopez et al., 2005).

Another study reported that significantly reduced rates of preterm births and low birth weight infants were observed for pregnant women who received plaque control instructions and scaling and root planing (Tarannum and Faizuddin, 2007). A three-year retrospective examination of a large insurance company database suggested that receiving preventive dental treatment is associated with a lower incidence of adverse birth outcomes compared with instances in which no dental services are delivered (Albert et al., 2011). However, a large multi-center study that included over 800 patients reported that periodontal treatment had no effect on pregnancy outcomes, recording the occurrence of preterm birth as 12% in the treatment group and 12.8% in the control group (Michalowicz et al., 2006).

Notably, the incidence of adverse birth outcomes from the various studies was lower among women who received some dental care and more so among those who received post-delivery periodontal care or those who received prophylactic treatment compared with those who received no dental care. The beneficial effect of dental care during the gestation period among these health-conscious and care-seeking women might also represent a coincidence. Good oral hygiene practices, however, can minimize gingival disease during pregnancy (Gibbs, 2001). Therefore, it has been recommended that all women should have a dental examination and appropriate dental hygiene care at least once during their pregnancy (Lieff et al., 2004). The American Academy of Periodontology recommends that women considering pregnancy or who are pregnant undergo a periodontal examination and receive the appropriate preventive and/or therapeutic services, if indicated.

8. Conclusions from the meta-analysis

The association between maternal periodontitis with adverse pregnancy outcomes such as low birthweight, pre-term birth and pre-eclampsia has been investigated for the past 20 years.

Several systematic reviews and meta-analysis has been conducted on various aspect of the association (Table 5). However, the strength of the observed associations based on clinical parameters is modest and seems to vary according to the population studied, the method used to assess periodontal diseases (Ide and Papapanou, 2013)

Khader and Ta'ani (2005) conducted a meta-analysis of periodontal disease in relation to the risk of preterm birth/low birth weight (PTB/LBW) based on two case-control studies and three prospective cohort studies. The sample sizes in the studies ranged from 80 to 1,313 women, with an age range between 12 and 40 years old. The odds ratio in these studies ranged from 3.5 to 7.5. Pregnant women with periodontal disease had an overall adjusted odds ratio of preterm birth that was 4.28 times higher than the odds ratio for healthy subjects (95% CI: 2.62 to 6.99; $P < 0.005$). They concluded that periodontal disease in pregnant mothers significantly increases the risk of subsequent preterm births or low birth weights.

Based on the meta-analysis, Xiong et al. (2006) concluded that periodontal disease might be associated with an increased risk of adverse pregnancy outcomes. They analyzed 44 studies (26 case-control studies, 13 cohort studies, and five controlled trials). The authors observed that the findings from observational studies yielded inconsistent conclusions on the relationship between periodontal disease and various pregnancy outcomes. Of the 39 observational studies, 25 studies (16 case-control and nine cohort) suggested that periodontal disease was associated with an increased risk of adverse pregnancy outcomes. Several studies demonstrated a direct relationship between the intensity of the periodontal disease and the risk of adverse pregnancy outcomes.

Vergnes and Sixou (2007) too echoed the same association when they reviewed 17 observational studies (11 case/controls, four cohorts, and two cross-sectionals) resulting in preterm low birth weight with an OR = 2.83 (95% CI: 1.95-4.10, P < 0.0001) and low birth weight with OR = 4.03 (95% CI: 2.05-7.93, P < 0.0001).

Though most of the studies have focused on the pregnancy outcome and periodontitis, very few studies have addressed the effect of periodontal treatment on adverse pregnancy outcome. One such review (Michalowicz et al., 2013) analyzed the same and resulted in a lone study on 303 Brazilian women 18 to 35 years of age with a gestational age ≤20 weeks. Randomization was stratified on smoking. All women, regardless of their periodontal status, received comprehensive non-surgical treatment (test group: oral hygiene instruction, scaling and root planing, and at least monthly follow-up visits) or supragingival scaling and oral hygiene instruction (control group).Despite statistically significant and substantial improvements in clinical periodontal measures with treatment (e.g. bleeding on probing (BOP) was reduced from 50% to 11%), there were no significant differences between test and control groups in preterm birth rates at <37 weeks (11.7 versus 9.1%, respectively, p = 0.57) or at <35 weeks (5.5% versus 5.8%, p = 0.99), or in fractions of infants weighing <2500 g (5.6% versus 4.1%,p = 0.59).

In a meta-analysis of the seven randomized trials, Polyzos and colleagues (2009) summarized that overall treatment of periodontal problems substantially reduced the rate of preterm delivery. They evaluated seven randomized controlled trials (n=2,663). There was a statistically significant reduction in incidence of preterm birth (OR 0.55, 95% CI 0.35 to 0.86, p<0.05) and low birth weight (OR 0.48, 95% CI 0.23 to 1.00, p<0.05) in women who received periodontal treatment compared to those who did not. The review findings suggested that treatment of periodontal disease during pregnancy reduced the rate of preterm birth and may reduce the incidence of low birth weight in infants.

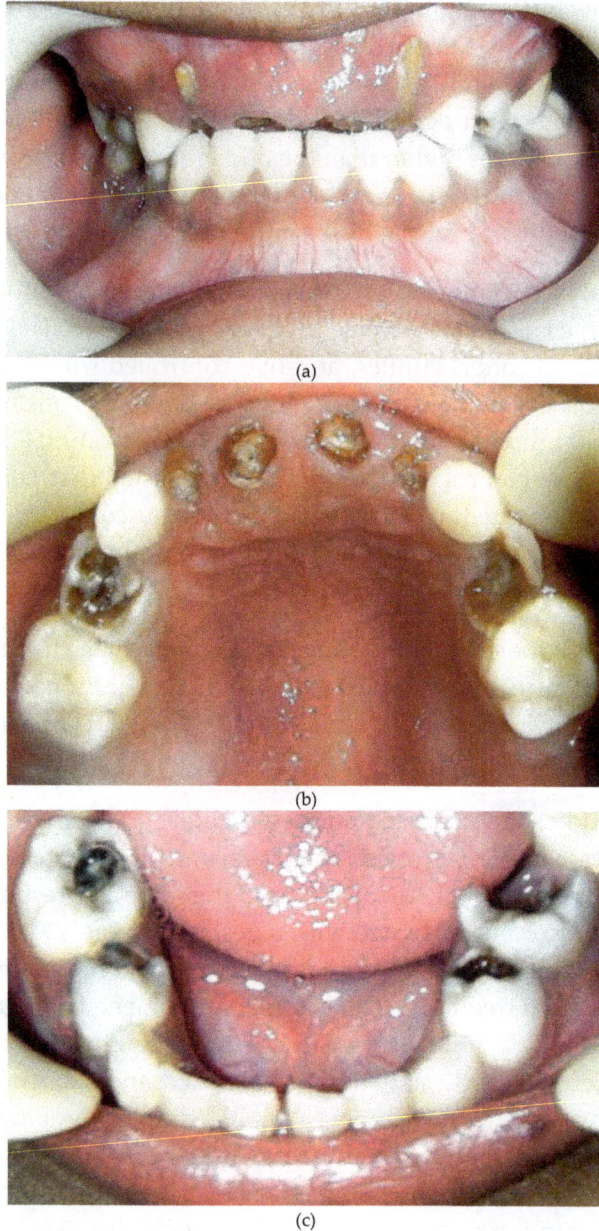

(a)

(b)

(c)

Figure 2. Early childhood caries

Polyzos et al (2010) examined whether treatment of periodontal disease with scaling and root planing during pregnancy is associated with a reduction in the preterm birth rate in randomized controlled trials. Of the 11 trials (with 6558 women), five trials were considered to be of high methodological quality (low risk of bias), whereas the rest were low quality (high or unclear risk of bias). It is noteworthy to see that the results among low and high quality trials were consistently diverse; low quality trials supported a beneficial effect of treatment, and high quality trials provided clear evidence that no such effect exists (odds ratio 1.15, 95% confidence interval 0.95 to 1.40; P=0.15).

9. Maternal oral health and early childhood caries

Early childhood caries (ECC) is an infectious disease that can present as soon as an infant's teeth erupt. ECC can progress rapidly and may have a lasting detrimental impact on the health and well-being of the child. Mothers with poor oral health and high levels of cariogenic oral bacteria are at greater risk for infecting their children with bacteria and increasing the risk of their children developing caries at an early age (Ramos-Gomez et al., 2002). *Streptococcus mutans* (MS) colonization of an infant may occur from the time of birth (Berkowitz, 2006), and significant colonization occurs after dental eruption, as the teeth provide non-shedding and other surfaces for adherence. (Wan et al., 2001; Tanner et al., 2002).

Cariogenic bacteria can be transmitted from mother to child by behaviors that directly pass saliva such as sharing a spoon when tasting baby food, cleaning a dropped pacifier by mouth or wiping the baby's mouth with saliva (Berkowitz, 2003). Reducing the transmission of cariogenic bacteria can be accomplished by reducing the maternal reservoir, avoiding vectors, and increasing the child's resistance to colonization (Li et al., 2003). Studies have demonstrated the effectiveness of a primary prevention program initiated during pregnancy to significantly improve the oral health of mothers and their children (Gunay et al., 1998; Soderling et al., 2001). Hence, comprehensive dental care for pregnant women is imperative to safeguard their oral and general health, as well as to reduce their children's caries risk (Brambilla et al., 1998; Boggess and Edelstein, 2006).

10. Gingival overgrowth related to pregnancy

Hormonal changes during pregnancy have been associated with varying types of gingival enlargement. These changes can potentiate the effects of local irritants on gingival connective tissue. Localized gingival overgrowth (pregnancy gingival tumor) is found in 0.2-0.5% of pregnant females. It occurs as a benign, rapidly growing lesion, usually in the 1st trimester of pregnancy and extending up to 3rd trimester. A pregnancy gingival tumor is a smooth or lobulated exophytic lesion with a pedunculated or sessile base (Srivastava et al., 2013) (Figure 3.). Several theories and speculations have been suggested to explain its occurrence during pregnancy, and meticulous maintenance of oral hygiene during pregnancy is important in reducing its incidence and the severity of gingival inflammation. Hormonal factors might play a role in aggravating gingivitis and gingival overgrowth (Oettinger-Barak et al., 2006; Andrikopoulou et al., 2013)

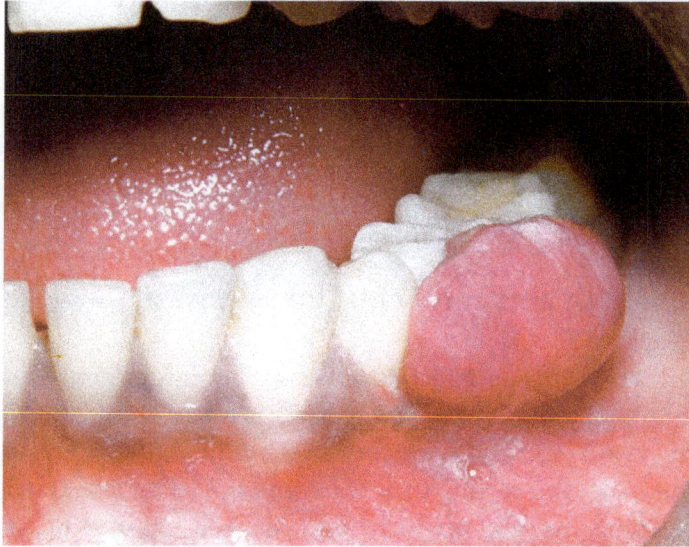

Figure 3. Pregnancy gingival overgrowth

11. Conclusion

Birth weight is considered to be an important determinant of the chances that an infant survives, grows, and matures. Maternal risk factors include age, height, weight, socio-economic status, ethnicity, smoking, alcohol use, nutritional status, and stress (Copper et al., 1996; Davenport et al., 2002). A review of the available literature has shown an association between periodontal disease and early pregnancy loss, preterm birth, low birth weight and preeclampsia (Jeffcoat et al., 2001; Gomes-Filho et al., 2007; Vergnes and Sixou, 2007; Xiong et al., 2007). However, the results regarding the treatment of oral disease during pregnancy are conflicting; some studies suggest a reduction in the rate of preterm births and dental caries (Brambilla et al., 1998; Jeffcoat et al., 2003; Lopez et al., 2005), whereas others show no impact (Michalowicz et al., 2006; Offenbacher et al., 2009; Macones et al., 2010).

The hypothesis that infection elsewhere in the body may influence PLBW has led to an increased awareness of the potential role of chronic bacterial infections. Periodontal disease is associated with a chronic Gram-negative infection of the periodontal tissues that results in a long-term local elevation of pro-inflammatory prostaglandins and cytokines and an increase in systemic levels of some of these inflammatory mediators (Page and Kornman, 1997). The evidence suggests that periodontitis can have a significant effect on systemic health. Periodontal disease is associated with many adverse pregnancy outcomes such as preterm delivery (Xiong et al., 2006), preeclampsia (Canakci et al., 2004), abortion and stillbirth (Moore et al., 2004), low birth weight (LBW) infants (Jarjoura et al., 2005) and preterm LBW infants (Xiong et al., 2006).

The strength of the association between periodontal disease and PTLB ranges from a two-fold to a seven-fold increase in risk. Although there are several data suggesting a relationship between maternal periodontal infection and preterm birth, several studies have failed to demonstrate such an association (Davenport et al., 2002; Holbrook et al., 2004; Moore et al., 2004; Buduneli et al., 2005; Rajapakse et al., 2005). Some of the factors that might have affected these observations are the lack of a consistent clinical definition and the failure to control for potential confounders (Holbrook et al., 2004; Moore et al., 2004; Buduneli et al., 2005). Another potential reason for the disparate findings among studies is the differences in the populations studied.

Several common risk factors are responsible for PLBW, such as age, socioeconomic status, and smoking, along with periodontal diseases. Because the inflammatory mediators that occur in periodontal diseases also play an important part in the initiation of labor, it is possible that a biological mechanism links the two conditions. Furthermore, intervention studies, animal studies, and more detailed mechanistic examinations are needed to directly correlate periodontal diseases to PLBW babies and eliminate the confounding effects of various other risk factors.

Author, year	Subjects, cases/ controls	Adverse pregnancy outcome	Periodontitis evaluation	Findings	Association
Jacob and Nath (2014), India	170/170	LBW	BOP, PD, CAL	Periodontitis represents a strong, independent, and clinically significant risk factor for LBW	Significant
Bulut et al. (2014), Turkey	50/50	PTB	PPD, CAL	The findings indicated that maternal periodontitis was not a possible risk factor for pre-term delivery	Significant
Santa Cruz et al. (2013), Spain	54/116	PTB	Microbiological tests	Clinical periodontal condition was not associated with adverse pregnancy outcomes in a Spanish Caucasian population with medium-high educational level	Non-significant
Kumar et al. (2013), India	61/132	LBW	Periodontal examination	Maternal periodontitis is associated with an increased preterm delivery and low birthweight infants.	Significant
Cruz et al (2009) Brazil	164/388	LBW	PI, BOP, PD, CAL	The findings suggest an association between periodontal disease and low birth weight among mothers with low education levels	Significant
Vettore et al. (2008)	150/66	PTB / LBW	PI, CI, BOP, PD, CAL	PD was significantly higher in non-preterm low birth weight controls than in subjects in the preterm low birthweight.	Non-significant

Author, year	Subjects, cases/ controls	Adverse pregnancy outcome	Periodontitis evaluation	Findings	Association
Brazil					
Santo-Pereira (2007) Brazil	124	PTB	Periodontitis was classified based on CAL	Periodontal disease more prevalent in women with preterm vs. term labor	Significant
Bassani et al. (2007), Brazil	304/611	LBW	PD, CAL	Similar rate of periodontal disease among cases and controls	Non-significant
Gomes-Filho et al. (2006), Brazil	44/177	PLBW	PI, PD, BOP, CAL	No statistically significant difference in the periodontal clinical parameters between the groups	Non-significant
Wood et al. (2006), Canada	50/101	PTB	Oral hygiene index simplified, PD, CAL, BOP	There was no difference in the proportion of sites with significant attachment loss.	Non-significant
Skuldbol et al. (2006), Denmark	21/33	PTB	PI, PD, BOP, Bitewing radiographs	No association between periodontal disease and preterm birth was found	Non-significant
Radnai et al. (2006), Hungary	77/84	PTB	PI, CI, BOP, PD	A significant association was found between PB and initial chronic localized periodontitis	Significant
Bosnjak et al. (2006), Croatia	17/64	PTB	CAL, PD, Papillary bleeding index	Periodontal disease was a significant independent risk factor for PTB.	Significant
Alves and Ribeiro (2006), Brazil	19/40	PLBW	The periodontal screening and recording	There was a higher rate of periodontal disease in cases (84.21%-16/19) as compared with controls (37.5% -15/40).	Significant
Moore et al. (2005) UK	61/93 (154)	PTB	PI, PD, CAL, BOP	No association between periodontal disease and pregnancy outcome	Non-significant
Noack et al. (2005), Germany	59/42	PLBW	PI, BOP, PD, CAL	Periodontitis was not a detectable risk factor for preterm low birth weight.	Non-significant
Buduneli et al. (2005) Turkey	53/128 (181)	PTB/LBW	BOP, PD, PI	No difference in periodontal disease between cases and controls	Non-significant
Jarjoura et al. (2005) USA	83/120 (203)	PTB/LBW	PI, BOP, PD, CAL	Periodontal disease associated with PTB/LBW	Significant

Author, year	Subjects, cases/ controls	Adverse pregnancy outcome	Periodontitis evaluation	Findings	Association
Moliterno et al. (2005), Brazil	76/75	PLBW	PD, CAL	Significant associations with low birth weight babies was periodontitis	Significant
Moore et al. (2004), UK	48/82	PTB	PI, PD, CAL, BOP	No statistically significant difference in the carriage of the IL-1P + [3953] allelic variant between cases and controls	Non-significant
Goepfert et al. (2004) USA	95/44	PTB	CAL	Multivariable analyses supported the association between severe periodontal disease and spontaneous preterm birth.	Significant
Mokeem et al. (2004) Saudi Arabia	30/60	PLBW	PD, BOP, CI, CPITN,	There is a correlation between periodontal disease and PLBW	Significant
Radnai et al. (2004)Hungary	41/44	PTB /LBW	PD,BOP ,CI	Periodontitis can be regarded as an important risk factor for PTB	Significant
Davenport et al. (2002) UK	236/507(743)	PLBW	PD, BOP, CPITN	No evidence for an association between periodontal disease and PLBW.	Non-significant
Louro et al. (2001)Brazil	13/13	LBW	Extension and severity index	Periodontal disease may be a risk factor for LBW	Significant
Dasanayake et al. (2001) USA	17/63	LBW	*Porphyromonas gingivalis (P.g)*, Serum IgG levels	Women with higher levels of P.g. IgG had higher odds of giving birth to LBW infants	Significant
Sembene et al (2000). Senegal	26/87	LBW	CPITN score: <1 1- 1.99 2- 2.99 "/>3	Periodontal disease is a potential risk factor for LBW	Significant
Dasanayake et al(1998) Thailand	50/ 50	LBW	DMFT and CPITN	Periodontal disease associated with LBW	Significant
Offenbacher et al. (1996) USA	93/31	PTB/LBW	CAL	Periodontal disease associated with PTB/LBW	Significant

PTB- Preterm Birth; PLBW- Preterm Low Birthweight; LBW- Low Birth Weight; PI-Plaque Index; GI- Gingival Index ; PD- Probing Depth; CAL- Clinical Attachment Level; CI calculus index; BOP- Bleeding On Probing; CAL - Clinical Attachment Level; CPITN- Community Periodontal Index for Treatment Needs ; DMFT - Decayed, Missing, and Filled Teeth

Table 1. Case-control studies on the relationship between adverse pregnancy outcome and periodontal disease

Study/Country	Sample size	Periodontal disease - Parameters	Conclusions	Association
Muwazi et al (2014)	400	PPD, BOP,CD GR, CPI	Significant association only between gingival recession and low birth weight	Significant
Kothiwale et al (2014)	770	PPD , CPI	The severity of periodontal disease was associated with an increased rate of pre-term infants. Severe anemia and periodontal infection may have an adverse effect on pregnancy and fetal development.	Significant
Ammanagi (2014) India	290	Not Known	Periodontal disease is a risk factor for PLBW	Significant
Abati et al (2013) Italy	750	Comprehensive oral and dental examination	Data failed to demonstrate the association between periodontitis and preterm birth and low birth weight.	Non - significant
Srinivas et al. (2009) India	786	CAL	No association between Periodontal disease and Pre term birth	Non - significant
Agueda et al. (2008) Spain	1200	PD,CAL,BOP	No significant association between periodontitis and low birth weight	Non - significant
Mobeen et al. (2008) Pakistan	1152	PD, CAL,PI, GI	Preterm birth and low birthweight were not related to measures of periodontal disease.	Non - significant
Pitiphat et al. (2008) USA	1635	Self-reported periodontitis Radiographs	The results suggest that periodontitis is an independent risk factor for poor pregnancy outcome among middle-class women.	Significant
Sharma et al. (2007) Fiji Islands	670	CPITN	There is a highly significant association between pre-term birth and moderate to severe periodontal disease	Significant
Toygar et al., (2007) Turkey	3576	CPITN	Maternal periodontal disease may be a risk factor for PTB and LBW	Significant
Rajapakse et al (2005) Sri Lanka	227	PI,CAL,BOP	Suggestive association between pre term low birth weight and periodontitis	Significant
Dortbudak et al. (2005) Austria	36	PD	Periodontitis can induce a primary host response in chorioamnnion leading to PTB	Significant
Moore et al (2004) UK	3738	PI,CAL,BOP,PD	No association between either PTB or LBW and periodontal disease.	Not Significant
Holbrook et al. (2004)	96	PD, gingival culture	No link between low grade periodontal disease and PTB	Not Significant

Study/Country	Sample size	Periodontal disease - Parameters	Conclusions	Association
Iceland				
Romero et al (2002) Venezuela	69	PI- Russell's Index	Periodontal disease is a risk factor for PTB &LBW	Significant
Lopez et al (2002) Chile	639	PD,CAL	Periodontal disease is an independent risk factor for PTB and LBW	Significant
Offenbacher et al (2001) USA	767	PD, CAL	Periodontal disease is a risk factor for PTB and LBW	Significant
Jeffcoat et al. (2001) USA	1313	CAL, PD	Periodontal disease is an independent risk for PTB	Significant

PTB- Preterm Birth; PLBW- Preterm Low Birthweight; LBW- Low Birth Weight; PI-Plaque Index; GI- Gingival Index ; PD- Probing Depth; CAL- Clinical Attachment Level; CI calculus index; BOP- Bleeding On Probing; PI - Periodontal Index ; CAL - Clinical Attachment Level; PPD-Probing Pocket Depth; CD - Calculus Deposit; CPI- Community Periodontal Index

Table 2. Adverse outcomes of pregnancy, pregnancy : Pre term birth weight/ low birth weight and Pre term weight-Cohort Studies

Author, year, country	Subjects, cases/controls	Periodontitis evaluation	Observations	Association
Kumar et al. (2013) India	61/132	PI,CAL,BOP	Maternal periodontitis is associated with an increased risk of pre-eclampsia.	Significant
Chaparro et al (2013) Chile	43/11	PI,CAL,BOP	Increased IL-6 levels in GCF in early pregnancy were associated with increased preeclampsia risk.	Significant
Taghzouti et al (2012) Canada	92/245	CAL,PD	No association between periodontal disease and preeclampsia	Significant
Hirano et al. (2012) Japan	18/109	PI,CAL,BOP	No statistically significant association between preeclampsia and periodontitis.	Not Significant
Wang et al. (2012) Japan	13/106	CAL	Polymorphism and subgingival DNA level of A. actinomycetemcomitans were significantly associated with preeclampsia.	Significant
Ha et al. (2011) Korea	16/48	CAL	Periodontal disease could be associated with preeclampsia	Significant
Politano et al (2011) Brazil	58/58	CAL,BOP,PD	There was an association between preeclampsia and periodontitis	Significant

Author, year, country	Subjects, cases/controls	Periodontitis evaluation	Observations	Association
Shetty et al. (2010) India	30/100	PD,CAL,GI	Periodontitis both at enrolment (OR = 5.78, 95% CI 2.41-13.89) as well as within 48 hours of delivery (OR = 20.15, 95% CI 4.55-89.29), may be associated with an increased risk of preeclampsia.	Significant
Nabet et al. (2010) France	1108/1094	CAL.PD,BOP	Maternal periodontitis is associated with an increased risk of induced preterm birth due to pre-eclampsia.	Significant
Lohsoonthorn et al. (2009) Thailand	150/150	PD,CAL	No association between periodontal disease and preeclampsia	Not Significant
Srinivas et al (2009) India	786	CAL	No association between periodontitis and pre-eclampsia	Not Significant
Siqueira et al.(2008) Brazil	164/1042	PD,CAL,BOP	Maternal periodontitis is a risk factor associated with preeclampsia.	Significant
Canakci et al (Canakci et al., 2007) Turkey	38/21	PD, CAL, BOP	Mild to severe periodontal disease is associated with an increased risk for development of preeclampsia	Significant
Kunnen et al (2007) Netherlands	17/35	PI, CI, BOP, R, PD	Severe periodontal disease was associated with increase of early onset preeclampsia	Significant
Barak et al (2007) Israel	16/14		Women with preeclampsia had higher prevalence of periopathogenic in bacterial placental tissue than controls	Significant
Contreas et al (2006) Columbia	130/243	PD, CAL	Periodontal disease is associated with an increased risk for development of preeclampsia	Significant
Cota et al (2006) Brazil	109/479	PI, CI, BOP, R, PD	Periodontal disease is associated with an increased risk for development of preeclampsia	Significant
Khader et al (2006) Jordan	115/230	PD, CAL,PI,CI	No association between periodontal disease and preeclampsia	Significant
Oettinger et al. (2005) Israel	15/15	PD, CAL,PI,CI	Periodontal disease is associated with an increased risk for development of preeclampsia	Significant

Author, year, country	Subjects, cases/controls	Periodontitis evaluation	Observations	Association
Canakci et al. (2004) Turkey	41/41	PD, CAL, BOP	Periodontal disease is associated with an increased risk for development of preeclampsia	Significant
Castaldi et al (2006) Argentina	1562	CAL, PD	No association between periodontal disease and preeclampsia	Not significant
Boggess et al (2003) USA	763	PI,CAL,BOP, PD	Association between periodontal disease and preeclampsia	Significant

CAL- Clinical Attachment Level; PTB- Preterm Birth; PLBW- Preterm Low Birthweight; LBW- Low Birth Weight; PD-Probing Depth; BOP- Bleeding On Probing; CAL - Clinical Attachment Level; PPD-Probing Pocket Depth; CD - Calculus Deposit; CPI- Community Periodontal Index

Table 3. The relationship between periodontal disease and Preeclampsia : Observational studies

Author, year	Subjects cases/controls	Adverse pregnancy outcome	Type of Periodontal Therapy/intervention	Results
Albert (2011)	464/12321	LBW,PTB	Periodontal treatment	Significant
Tarannum and Faizuddin (2007)	53/68	PTB, LBW	Scaling and root planning (SRP) and Plaque control instructions	Significant
Michalowicz et al.(2006)	413/410	PTB, LBW	Scaling and oral hygiene instructions	Non-significant
Offenbacher et al.(2006)	40/34	PTB	SRP and advised to use of a sonic toothbrush	Significant
Sadatmansouri et al. (2006)	30/30	PLBW	Oral hygiene instructions, 0.2% Chlorhexidine mouth	Significant
Lopez et al.(2005)	580/290	PLBW	Scaling, Plaque control, 0.12% chlorhexidine	Significant
Jeffcoat et al. (2003)	366/723	PTB	Scaling and root planning	Significant
Lopez et al.(2002)	163/188	PLBW	scaling and root planing (SRP) and Oral Hygiene instructions	Significant
Mitchell-Lewis et al (2001)	74/ 90	PLBW	Oral prophylaxis	Significant

PTB- Preterm Birth; PLBW- Preterm Low Birthweight; LBW- Low Birth Weight

Table 4. Studies showing the relationship of periodontal therapy on preventing adverse pregnancy outcomes

Authors	Studies included	Outcomes	Conclusions
Ide and Papapanou (2013)	Cross-sectional, case-control or prospective cohort epidemiological studies on the association between periodontal status and preterm birth, low birthweight (LBW) or preeclampsia.Preterm birth (<37 weeks gestation), LBW (<2500 g), gestational age, small for gestational age, birthweight, pregnancy loss or miscarriage, or pre-eclampsia.	Although significant associations emerge from case-control and cross-sectional studies using periodontitis "case definitions," these were substantially attenuated in studies assessing periodontitis as a continuous variable.	Maternal periodontitis is modestly but significantly associated with LBW and preterm birth, but the definition of periodontitis appears to impact the findings. Data from prospective studies followed a similar pattern, but associations were generally weaker. Maternal periodontitis was significantly associated with pre-eclampsia. It is suggested that future studies employ both continuous and categorical assessments of periodontal status. Further use of the composite outcome preterm LBW is not encouraged.
Michalowicz et al. (2013)	To identify randomized controlled trials (RCTs) published between January 2011 and July 2012 and discuss all published RCTs testing whether periodontal therapy reduces rates of preterm birth and low birthweight.	The single RCT identified showed no significant effect of periodontal treatment on birth outcomes.	Non-surgical periodontal therapy, scaling and root planing, does not improve birth outcomes in pregnant women with periodontitis.
Polyzos et al. (2010)	11 Case control studies trials (with 6558 women)	Periodontal treatment had no significant effect on the overall rate of preterm birth (odds ratio 1.15, 95% confidence interval 0.95 to 1.40; P=0.15).Furthermore, treatment did not reduce the rate of low birthweight infants (odds ratio 1.07, 0.85 to 1.36;P=0.55).	Treatment of periodontal disease with scaling and root planing during pregnancy does not reduce the risk of preterm birth and should not be routinely recommended as a measure to prevent preterm birth
Polyzos et al (2009)	Seven randomized trials were included based on the criteria.There were 2663 patients: 1491 had been randomized to receive periodontal treatment and 1172 to no treatment.	Treatment resulted in significantly lower PTB (odds ratio [OR], 0.55; 95% confidence interval [CI], 0.350.86; P = .008) and borderline significantly lower LBW (OR, 0.48; 95% CI, 0.23-1.00;P = .049), whereas no difference was found for spontaneous abortion/stillbirth (OR, 0.73; 95% CI, 0.41-1.31; P = .292).	The analysis showed that treatment with scaling and/or root planing during pregnancy significantly reduces the rate of PTB and may reduce the rate of LBW infants.
Vergnes and Sixou (2007)	17 observational studies (11 case/controls, four cohorts, and two cross-sectionals)	Preterm low birth weight:OR = 2.83 (95% CI: 1.95-4.10, P < 0.0001)LBW:	These findings indicate a likely association, but it needs to be

Authors	Studies included	Outcomes	Conclusions
		OR = 4.03 (95% CI: 2.05-7.93, P < 0.0001)	confirmed by large, well- designed, multicenter trials
Xiong et al. (2006)	44 studies (26 case-control studies, 13 cohort studies, and five controlled trials)	Twenty nine suggested an association between periodontal disease and increased risk of adverse pregnancy outcome (ORs ranging from 1.10 to 20.0) and 15 found no evidence of an association (ORs ranging from 0.78 to 2.54) Preterm Low birth weight:RR = 0.53, 95% CI: 0.30-0.95, P < 0.05Preterm birth: RR = 0.79, 95% CI: 0.55-1.11, P "/> 0.05 Low birth weight: RR = 0.86, 95% CI: 0.58%1.29, P "/> 0.05	The published literature is not vigorous to clinically link periodontal disease and/or its treatment to specific adverse pregnancy outcomes
Khader and Ta'ani (2005)	5 studies (two case-control and three prospective cohorts)	PTB: OR = 4.28 (95% CI: 2.62-6.99; P < 0.005)PTLBW: OR = 5.28 (95% CI: 2.21-12.62; P < 0.005)Either PTB or LBW: OR = 2.30 (95% CI: 1.21-4.38; P < 0.005)	Periodontal diseases in the pregnant mother significantly increase the risk of subsequent preterm birth or low birth weight

PTB- Preterm Birth; PLBW- Preterm Low Birthweight; LBW- Low Birth Weight; PI-Plaque Index; GI- Gingival Index ; PD- Probing Depth; CAL- Clinical Attachment Level; CI calculus index; BOP- Bleeding On Probing; PI - Periodontal Index ; CAL - Clinical Attachment Level; PPD-Probing Pocket Depth; CD - Calculus Deposit; CPI- Community Periodontal Index ;

Table 5. Meta-analysis on periodontal disease and adverse pregnancy outcomes

Author details

Sukumaran Anil[1]*, Raed M. Alrowis[1], Elna P. Chalisserry[2], Vemina P. Chalissery[3], Hani S. AlMoharib[1] and Asala F. Al-Sulaimani[4]

*Address all correspondence to: drsanil@gmail.com

1 Department of Periodontics and Community Dentistry, College of Dentistry, King Saud University, Riyadh, Saudi Arabia

2 College of Dentistry, King Saud University, Riyadh, Saudi Arabia

3 Mahatma Gandhi Dental College and Hospital, Jaipur, Rajasthan, India

4 King Saud University, Riyadh, Saudi Arabia

References

[1]   Abati S, Villa A, Cetin I, Dessole S, Luglie PF, Strohmenger L, Ottolenghi L, Campus GG. 2013. Lack of association between maternal periodontal status and adverse pregnancy outcomes: a multicentric epidemiologic study. The journal of maternal-fetal & neonatal medicine : the official journal of the European Association of Perinatal Medicine, the Federation of Asia and Oceania Perinatal Societies, the International Society of Perinatal Obstet 26:369-372.

[2]   Agueda A, Ramon JM, Manau C, Guerrero A, Echeverria JJ. 2008. Periodontal disease as a risk factor for adverse pregnancy outcomes: a prospective cohort study. Journal of clinical periodontology 35:16-22.

[3]   Albert DA, Begg MD, Andrews HF, Williams SZ, Ward A, Conicella ML, Rauh V, Thomson JL, Papapanou PN. 2011. An examination of periodontal treatment, dental care, and pregnancy outcomes in an insured population in the United States. American journal of public health 101:151-156.

[4]   Alves RT, Ribeiro RA. 2006. Relationship between maternal periodontal disease and birth of preterm low weight babies. Brazilian oral research 20:318-323.

[5]   Ammanagi R. 2014. Low birth weight among newborns and maternal poor periodontal status. Indian journal of public health 58:69.

[6]   Andrikopoulou M, Chatzistamou I, Gkilas H, Vilaras G, Sklavounou A. 2013. Assessment of angiogenic markers and female sex hormone receptors in pregnancy tumor of the gingiva. Journal of oral and maxillofacial surgery : official journal of the American Association of Oral and Maxillofacial Surgeons 71:1376-1381.

[7]   Barak S, Oettinger-Barak O, Machtei EE, Sprecher H, Ohel G. 2007. Evidence of periopathogenic microorganisms in placentas of women with preeclampsia. Journal of periodontology 78:670-676.

[8]   Barak S, Oettinger-Barak O, Oettinger M, Machtei EE, Peled M, Ohel G. 2003. Common oral manifestations during pregnancy: a review. Obstetrical & gynecological survey 58:624-628.

[9]   Bassani DG, Olinto MT, Kreiger N. 2007. Periodontal disease and perinatal outcomes: a case-control study. Journal of clinical periodontology 34:31-39.

[10] Berkowitz RJ. 2003. Causes, treatment and prevention of early childhood caries: a microbiologic perspective. Journal 69:304-307.

[11] Berkowitz RJ. 2006. Mutans streptococci: acquisition and transmission. Pediatric dentistry 28:106-109; discussion 192-108.

[12] Boggess KA, Beck JD, Murtha AP, Moss K, Offenbacher S. 2006. Maternal periodontal disease in early pregnancy and risk for a small-for-gestational-age infant. American journal of obstetrics and gynecology 194:1316-1322.

[13] Boggess KA, Edelstein BL. 2006. Oral health in women during preconception and pregnancy: implications for birth outcomes and infant oral health. Maternal and child health journal 10:S169-174.

[14] Boggess KA, Lieff S, Murtha AP, Moss K, Beck J, Offenbacher S. 2003. Maternal periodontal disease is associated with an increased risk for preeclampsia. Obstetrics and gynecology 101:227-231.

[15] Boggess KA, Madianos PN, Preisser JS, Moise KJ, Jr., Offenbacher S. 2005. Chronic maternal and fetal Porphyromonas gingivalis exposure during pregnancy in rabbits. American journal of obstetrics and gynecology 192:554-557.

[16] Bosnjak A, Relja T, Vucicevic-Boras V, Plasaj H, Plancak D. 2006. Pre-term delivery and periodontal disease: a case-control study from Croatia. Journal of clinical periodontology 33:710-716.

[17] Brambilla E, Felloni A, Gagliani M, Malerba A, Garcia-Godoy F, Strohmenger L. 1998. Caries prevention during pregnancy: results of a 30-month study. Journal of the American Dental Association 129:871-877.

[18] Buduneli N, Baylas H, Buduneli E, Turkoglu O, Kose T, Dahlen G. 2005. Periodontal infections and pre-term low birth weight: a case-control study. Journal of clinical periodontology 32:174-181.

[19] Buduneli N, Kinane DF. 2011. Host-derived diagnostic markers related to soft tissue destruction and bone degradation in periodontitis. Journal of clinical periodontology 38 Suppl 11:85-105.

[20] Bulut G, Olukman O, Calkavur S. 2014. Is there a relationship between maternal periodontitis and pre-term birth? A prospective hospital-based case-control study. Acta odontologica Scandinavica:1-8.

[21] Canakci V, Canakci CF, Canakci H, Canakci E, Cicek Y, Ingec M, Ozgoz M, Demir T, Dilsiz A, Yagiz H. 2004. Periodontal disease as a risk factor for pre-eclampsia: a case control study. The Australian & New Zealand journal of obstetrics & gynaecology 44:568-573.

[22] Canakci V, Canakci CF, Yildirim A, Ingec M, Eltas A, Erturk A. 2007. Periodontal disease increases the risk of severe pre-eclampsia among pregnant women. Journal of clinical periodontology 34:639-645.

[23] Castaldi JL, Bertin MS, Gimenez F, Lede R. 2006. [Periodontal disease: Is it a risk factor for premature labor, low birth weight or preeclampsia?]. Rev Panam Salud Publica 19:253-258.

[24] Chaparro A, Sanz A, Quintero A, Inostroza C, Ramirez V, Carrion F, Figueroa F, Serra R, Illanes SE. 2013. Increased inflammatory biomarkers in early pregnancy is associated with the development of pre-eclampsia in patients with periodontitis: a case control study. Journal of periodontal research 48:302-307.

[25] Contreras A, Herrera JA, Soto JE, Arce RM, Jaramillo A, Botero JE. 2006. Periodontitis is associated with preeclampsia in pregnant women. Journal of periodontology 77:182-188.

[26] Copper RL, Goldenberg RL, Das A, Elder N, Swain M, Norman G, Ramsey R, Cotroneo P, Collins BA, Johnson F, Jones P, Meier AM. 1996. The preterm prediction study: maternal stress is associated with spontaneous preterm birth at less than thirty-five weeks' gestation. National Institute of Child Health and Human Development Maternal-Fetal Medicine Units Network. American journal of obstetrics and gynecology 175:1286-1292.

[27] Cota LO, Guimaraes AN, Costa JE, Lorentz TC, Costa FO. 2006. Association between maternal periodontitis and an increased risk of preeclampsia. Journal of periodontology 77:2063-2069.

[28] Cruz SS, Costa Mda C, Gomes-Filho IS, Rezende EJ, Barreto ML, Dos Santos CA, Vianna MI, Passos JS, Cerqueira EM. 2009. Contribution of periodontal disease in pregnant women as a risk factor for low birth weight. Community dentistry and oral epidemiology 37:527-533.

[29] Cruz SS, Costa Mda C, Gomes Filho IS, Vianna MI, Santos CT. 2005. [Maternal periodontal disease as a factor associated with low birth weight]. Revista de saude publica 39:782-787.

[30] Darveau RP, Tanner A, Page RC. 1997. The microbial challenge in periodontitis. Periodontology 2000 14:12-32.

[31] Dasanayake AP. 1998. Poor periodontal health of the pregnant woman as a risk factor for low birth weight. Annals of periodontology / the American Academy of Periodontology 3:206-212.

[32] Dasanayake AP, Boyd D, Madianos PN, Offenbacher S, Hills E. 2001. The association between Porphyromonas gingivalis-specific maternal serum IgG and low birth weight. Journal of periodontology 72:1491-1497.

[33] Davenport ES, Williams CE, Sterne JA, Murad S, Sivapathasundram V, Curtis MA. 2002. Maternal periodontal disease and preterm low birthweight: case-control study. Journal of dental research 81:313-318.

[34] Dortbudak O, Eberhardt R, Ulm M, Persson GR. 2005. Periodontitis, a marker of risk in pregnancy for preterm birth. Journal of clinical periodontology 32:45-52.

[35] Duarte PM, da Rocha M, Sampaio E, Mestnik MJ, Feres M, Figueiredo LC, Bastos MF, Faveri M. 2010. Serum levels of cytokines in subjects with generalized chronic

and aggressive periodontitis before and after non-surgical periodontal therapy: a pilot study. Journal of periodontology 81:1056-1063.

[36] Furugen R, Hayashida H, Yamaguchi N, Yoshihara A, Ogawa H, Miyazaki H, Saito T. 2008. The relationship between periodontal condition and serum levels of resistin and adiponectin in elderly Japanese. Journal of periodontal research 43:556-562.

[37] Gibbs RS. 2001. The relationship between infections and adverse pregnancy outcomes: an overview. Annals of periodontology / the American Academy of Periodontology 6:153-163.

[38] Goepfert AR, Jeffcoat MK, Andrews WW, Faye-Petersen O, Cliver SP, Goldenberg RL, Hauth JC. 2004. Periodontal disease and upper genital tract inflammation in early spontaneous preterm birth. Obstetrics and gynecology 104:777-783.

[39] Goldenberg RL, Culhane JF, Iams JD, Romero R. 2008. Epidemiology and causes of preterm birth. Lancet 371:75-84.

[40] Goldenberg RL, Hauth JC, Andrews WW. 2000. Intrauterine infection and preterm delivery. The New England journal of medicine 342:1500-1507.

[41] Gomes-Filho IS, Cruz SS, Rezende EJ, Dos Santos CA, Soledade KR, Magalhaes MA, de Azevedo AC, Trindade SC, Vianna MI, Passos Jde S, Cerqueira EM. 2007. Exposure measurement in the association between periodontal disease and prematurity/low birth weight. Journal of clinical periodontology 34:957-963.

[42] Gomes-Filho IS, da Cruz SS, Rezende EJ, da Silveira BB, Trindade SC, Passos JS, de Freitas CO, Cerqueira EM, de Souza Teles Santos CA. 2006. Periodontal status as predictor of prematurity and low birth weight. J Public Health Dent 66:295-298.

[43] Gunay H, Dmoch-Bockhorn K, Gunay Y, Geurtsen W. 1998. Effect on caries experience of a long-term preventive program for mothers and children starting during pregnancy. Clinical oral investigations 2:137-142.

[44] Ha JE, Oh KJ, Yang HJ, Jun JK, Jin BH, Paik DI, Bae KH. 2011. Oral health behaviors, periodontal disease, and pathogens in preeclampsia: a case-control study in Korea. Journal of periodontology 82:1685-1692.

[45] Han YW. 2011. Oral health and adverse pregnancy outcomes - what's next? Journal of dental research 90:289-293.

[46] Han YW, Redline RW, Li M, Yin L, Hill GB, McCormick TS. 2004. Fusobacterium nucleatum induces premature and term stillbirths in pregnant mice: implication of oral bacteria in preterm birth. Infection and immunity 72:2272-2279.

[47] Hillier SL, Martius J, Krohn M, Kiviat N, Holmes KK, Eschenbach DA. 1988. A case-control study of chorioamnionic infection and histologic chorioamnionitis in prematurity. The New England journal of medicine 319:972-978.

[48] Hirano E, Sugita N, Kikuchi A, Shimada Y, Sasahara J, Iwanaga R, Tanaka K, Yoshie H. 2012. The association of Aggregatibacter actinomycetemcomitans with preeclamp-

sia in a subset of Japanese pregnant women. Journal of clinical periodontology 39:229-238.

[49] Holbrook WP, Oskarsdottir A, Fridjonsson T, Einarsson H, Hauksson A, Geirsson RT. 2004. No link between low-grade periodontal disease and preterm birth: a pilot study in a healthy Caucasian population. Acta odontologica Scandinavica 62:177-179.

[50] Ide M, Papapanou PN. 2013. Epidemiology of association between maternal periodontal disease and adverse pregnancy outcomes--systematic review. Journal of clinical periodontology 40 Suppl 14:S181-194.

[51] Jacob PS, Nath S. 2014. Periodontitis among poor rural Indian mothers increases the risk of low birth weight babies: a hospital-based case control study. Journal of periodontal & implant science 44:85-93.

[52] Jarjoura K, Devine PC, Perez-Delboy A, Herrera-Abreu M, D'Alton M, Papapanou PN. 2005. Markers of periodontal infection and preterm birth. American journal of obstetrics and gynecology 192:513-519.

[53] Jeffcoat MK, Geurs NC, Reddy MS, Cliver SP, Goldenberg RL, Hauth JC. 2001. Periodontal infection and preterm birth: results of a prospective study. Journal of the American Dental Association 132:875-880.

[54] Jeffcoat MK, Hauth JC, Geurs NC, Reddy MS, Cliver SP, Hodgkins PM, Goldenberg RL. 2003. Periodontal disease and preterm birth: results of a pilot intervention study. Journal of periodontology 74:1214-1218.

[55] Jensen J, Liljemark W, Bloomquist C. 1981. The effect of female sex hormones on subgingival plaque. Journal of periodontology 52:599-602.

[56] Khader YS, Jibreal M, Al-Omiri M, Amarin Z. 2006. Lack of association between periodontal parameters and preeclampsia. Journal of periodontology 77:1681-1687.

[57] Khader YS, Ta'ani Q. 2005. Periodontal diseases and the risk of preterm birth and low birth weight: a meta-analysis. Journal of periodontology 76:161-165.

[58] Kornman KS, Loesche WJ. 1980. The subgingival microbial flora during pregnancy. Journal of periodontal research 15:111-122.

[59] Kothiwale SV, Desai BR, Kothiwale VA, Gandhid M, Konin S. 2014. Periodontal disease as a potential risk factor for low birth weight and reduced maternal haemomglobin levels. Oral health & preventive dentistry 12:83-90.

[60] Kumar A, Basra M, Begum N, Rani V, Prasad S, Lamba AK, Verma M, Agarwal S, Sharma S. 2013. Association of maternal periodontal health with adverse pregnancy outcome. The journal of obstetrics and gynaecology research 39:40-45.

[61] Kunnen A, Blaauw J, van Doormaal JJ, van Pampus MG, van der Schans CP, Aarnoudse JG, van Winkelhoff AJ, Abbas F. 2007. Women with a recent history of early-

onset pre-eclampsia have a worse periodontal condition. Journal of clinical periodontology 34:202-207.

[62] Li Y, Dasanayake AP, Caufield PW, Elliott RR, Butts JT, 3rd. 2003. Characterization of maternal mutans streptococci transmission in an African American population. Dental clinics of North America 47:87-101.

[63] Lieff S, Boggess KA, Murtha AP, Jared H, Madianos PN, Moss K, Beck J, Offenbacher S. 2004. The oral conditions and pregnancy study: periodontal status of a cohort of pregnant women. Journal of periodontology 75:116-126.

[64] Lin D, Smith MA, Champagne C, Elter J, Beck J, Offenbacher S. 2003a. Porphyromonas gingivalis infection during pregnancy increases maternal tumor necrosis factor alpha, suppresses maternal interleukin-10, and enhances fetal growth restriction and resorption in mice. Infection and immunity 71:5156-5162.

[65] Lin D, Smith MA, Elter J, Champagne C, Downey CL, Beck J, Offenbacher S. 2003b. Porphyromonas gingivalis infection in pregnant mice is associated with placental dissemination, an increase in the placental Th1/Th2 cytokine ratio, and fetal growth restriction. Infection and immunity 71:5163-5168.

[66] Lohsoonthorn V, Kungsadalpipob K, Chanchareonsook P, Limpongsanurak S, Vanichjakvong O, Sutdhibhisal S, Sookprome C, Wongkittikraiwan N, Kamolpornwijit W, Jantarasaengaram S, Manotaya S, Siwawej V, Barlow WE, Fitzpatrick AL, Williams MA. 2009. Maternal periodontal disease and risk of preeclampsia: a case-control study. Am J Hypertens 22:457-463.

[67] Lopez NJ, Da Silva I, Ipinza J, Gutierrez J. 2005. Periodontal therapy reduces the rate of preterm low birth weight in women with pregnancy-associated gingivitis. Journal of periodontology 76:2144-2153.

[68] Lopez NJ, Smith PC, Gutierrez J. 2002. Periodontal therapy may reduce the risk of preterm low birth weight in women with periodontal disease: a randomized controlled trial. Journal of periodontology 73:911-924.

[69] Louro PM, Fiori HH, Filho PL, Steibel J, Fiori RM. 2001. [Periodontal disease in pregnancy and low birth weight]. J Pediatr (Rio J) 77:23-28.

[70] Macones GA, Parry S, Nelson DB, Strauss JF, Ludmir J, Cohen AW, Stamilio DM, Appleby D, Clothier B, Sammel MD, Jeffcoat M. 2010. Treatment of localized periodontal disease in pregnancy does not reduce the occurrence of preterm birth: results from the Periodontal Infections and Prematurity Study (PIPS). American journal of obstetrics and gynecology 202:147 e141-148.

[71] Madianos PN, Lieff S, Murtha AP, Boggess KA, Auten RL, Jr., Beck JD, Offenbacher S. 2001. Maternal periodontitis and prematurity. Part II: Maternal infection and fetal exposure. Annals of periodontology / the American Academy of Periodontology 6:175-182.

[72] Marakoglu I, Gursoy UK, Marakoglu K, Cakmak H, Ataoglu T. 2008. Periodontitis as a risk factor for preterm low birth weight. Yonsei medical journal 49:200-203.

[73] Mascarenhas P, Gapski R, Al-Shammari K, Wang HL. 2003. Influence of sex hormones on the periodontium. Journal of clinical periodontology 30:671-681.

[74] McGaw T. 2002. Periodontal disease and preterm delivery of low-birth-weight infants. Journal 68:165-169.

[75] Michalowicz BS, Gustafsson A, Thumbigere-Math V, Buhlin K. 2013. The effects of periodontal treatment on pregnancy outcomes. Journal of clinical periodontology 40 Suppl 14:S195-208.

[76] Michalowicz BS, Hodges JS, DiAngelis AJ, Lupo VR, Novak MJ, Ferguson JE, Buchanan W, Bofill J, Papapanou PN, Mitchell DA, Matseoane S, Tschida PA, Study OPT. 2006. Treatment of periodontal disease and the risk of preterm birth. The New England journal of medicine 355:1885-1894.

[77] Mitchell-Lewis D, Engebretson SP, Chen J, Lamster IB, Papapanou PN. 2001. Periodontal infections and pre-term birth: early findings from a cohort of young minority women in New York. Eur J Oral Sci 109:34-39.

[78] Mobeen N, Jehan I, Banday N, Moore J, McClure EM, Pasha O, Wright LL, Goldenberg RL. 2008. Periodontal disease and adverse birth outcomes: a study from Pakistan. American journal of obstetrics and gynecology 198:514 e511-518.

[79] Mokeem SA, Molla GN, Al-Jewair TS. 2004. The prevalence and relationship between periodontal disease and pre-term low birth weight infants at King Khalid University Hospital in Riyadh, Saudi Arabia. J Contemp Dent Pract 5:40-56.

[80] Moliterno LF, Monteiro B, Figueredo CM, Fischer RG. 2005. Association between periodontitis and low birth weight: a case-control study. Journal of clinical periodontology 32:886-890.

[81] Moore S, Ide M, Coward PY, Randhawa M, Borkowska E, Baylis R, Wilson RF. 2004. A prospective study to investigate the relationship between periodontal disease and adverse pregnancy outcome. British dental journal 197:251-258; discussion 247.

[82] Moore S, Randhawa M, Ide M. 2005. A case-control study to investigate an association between adverse pregnancy outcome and periodontal disease. Journal of clinical periodontology 32:1-5.

[83] Muwazi L, Rwenyonyi CM, Nkamba M, Kutesa A, Kagawa M, Mugyenyi G, Kwizera G, Okullo I. 2014. Periodontal conditions, low birth weight and preterm birth among postpartum mothers in two tertiary health facilities in Uganda. BMC oral health 14:42.

[84] Nabet C, Lelong N, Colombier ML, Sixou M, Musset AM, Goffinet F, Kaminski M, Epipap G. 2010. Maternal periodontitis and the causes of preterm birth: the case-control Epipap study. Journal of clinical periodontology 37:37-45.

[85] Noack B, Klingenberg J, Weigelt J, Hoffmann T. 2005. Periodontal status and preterm low birth weight: a case control study. Journal of periodontal research 40:339-345.

[86] Nordstrom ML, Cnattingius S. 1996. Effects on birthweights of maternal education, socio-economic status, and work-related characteristics. Scandinavian journal of social medicine 24:55-61.

[87] Oettinger-Barak O, Barak S, Ohel G, Oettinger M, Kreutzer H, Peled M, Machtei EE. 2005. Severe pregnancy complication (preeclampsia) is associated with greater periodontal destruction. Journal of periodontology 76:134-137.

[88] Oettinger-Barak O, Machtei EE, Ofer BI, Barak S, Peled M. 2006. Pregnancy tumor occurring twice in the same individual: report of a case and hormone receptors study. Quintessence international (Berlin, Germany : 1985) 37:213-218.

[89] Offenbacher S, Beck JD, Jared HL, Mauriello SM, Mendoza LC, Couper DJ, Stewart DD, Murtha AP, Cochran DL, Dudley DJ, Reddy MS, Geurs NC, Hauth JC, Maternal Oral Therapy to Reduce Obstetric Risk I. 2009. Effects of periodontal therapy on rate of preterm delivery: a randomized controlled trial. Obstetrics and gynecology 114:551-559.

[90] Offenbacher S, Katz V, Fertik G, Collins J, Boyd D, Maynor G, McKaig R, Beck J. 1996. Periodontal infection as a possible risk factor for preterm low birth weight. Journal of periodontology 67:1103-1113.

[91] Offenbacher S, Lieff S, Boggess KA, Murtha AP, Madianos PN, Champagne CM, McKaig RG, Jared HL, Mauriello SM, Auten RL, Jr., Herbert WN, Beck JD. 2001. Maternal periodontitis and prematurity. Part I: Obstetric outcome of prematurity and growth restriction. Annals of periodontology / the American Academy of Periodontology 6:164-174.

[92] Offenbacher S, Lin D, Strauss R, McKaig R, Irving J, Barros SP, Moss K, Barrow DA, Hefti A, Beck JD. 2006. Effects of periodontal therapy during pregnancy on periodontal status, biologic parameters, and pregnancy outcomes: a pilot study. Journal of periodontology 77:2011-2024.

[93] Page RC, Kornman KS. 1997. The pathogenesis of human periodontitis: an introduction. Periodontology 2000 14:9-11.

[94] Pitiphat W, Joshipura KJ, Gillman MW, Williams PL, Douglass CW, Rich-Edwards JW. 2008. Maternal periodontitis and adverse pregnancy outcomes. Community dentistry and oral epidemiology 36:3-11.

[95] Politano GT, Passini R, Nomura ML, Velloso L, Morari J, Couto E. 2011. Correlation between periodontal disease, inflammatory alterations and pre-eclampsia. Journal of periodontal research 46:505-511.

[96] Polyzos NP, Polyzos IP, Mauri D, Tzioras S, Tsappi M, Cortinovis I, Casazza G. 2009. Effect of periodontal disease treatment during pregnancy on preterm birth incidence: a metaanalysis of randomized trials. American journal of obstetrics and gynecology 200:225-232.

[97] Polyzos NP, Polyzos IP, Zavos A, Valachis A, Mauri D, Papanikolaou EG, Tzioras S, Weber D, Messinis IE. 2010. Obstetric outcomes after treatment of periodontal disease during pregnancy: systematic review and meta-analysis. Bmj 341:c7017.

[98] Radnai M, Gorzo I, Nagy E, Urban E, Novak T, Pal A. 2004. A possible association between preterm birth and early periodontitis. A pilot study. Journal of clinical periodontology 31:736-741.

[99] Radnai M, Gorzo I, Urban E, Eller J, Novak T, Pal A. 2006. Possible association between mother's periodontal status and preterm delivery. Journal of clinical periodontology 33:791-796.

[100] Rajapakse PS, Nagarathne M, Chandrasekra KB, Dasanayake AP. 2005. Periodontal disease and prematurity among non-smoking Sri Lankan women. Journal of dental research 84:274-277.

[101] Ramos-Gomez FJ, Weintraub JA, Gansky SA, Hoover CI, Featherstone JD. 2002. Bacterial, behavioral and environmental factors associated with early childhood caries. The Journal of clinical pediatric dentistry 26:165-173.

[102] Roberts JM, Pearson G, Cutler J, Lindheimer M, Pregnancy NWGoRoHD. 2003. Summary of the NHLBI Working Group on Research on Hypertension During Pregnancy. Hypertension 41:437-445.

[103] Romero BC, Chiquito CS, Elejalde LE, Bernardoni CB. 2002. Relationship between periodontal disease in pregnant women and the nutritional condition of their newborns. Journal of periodontology 73:1177-1183.

[104] Romero R, Espinoza J, Goncalves LF, Kusanovic JP, Friel LA, Nien JK. 2006. Inflammation in preterm and term labour and delivery. Seminars in fetal & neonatal medicine 11:317-326.

[105] Romero R, Mazor M, Sepulveda W, Avila C, Copeland D, Williams J. 1992. Tumor necrosis factor in preterm and term labor. American journal of obstetrics and gynecology 166:1576-1587.

[106] Sadatmansouri S, Sedighpoor N, Aghaloo M. 2006. Effects of periodontal treatment phase I on birth term and birth weight. Journal of the Indian Society of Pedodontics and Preventive Dentistry 24:23-26.

[107] Santa Cruz I, Herrera D, Martin C, Herrero A, Sanz M. 2013. Association between periodontal status and pre-term and/or low-birth weight in Spain: clinical and microbiological parameters. Journal of periodontal research 48:443-451.

[108] Santos-Pereira SA, Giraldo PC, Saba-Chujfi E, Amaral RL, Morais SS, Fachini AM, Goncalves AK. 2007. Chronic periodontitis and pre-term labour in Brazilian pregnant women: an association to be analysed. Journal of clinical periodontology 34:208-213.

[109] Sanz M, Kornman K, Working group 3 of joint EFPAAPw. 2013. Periodontitis and adverse pregnancy outcomes: consensus report of the Joint EFP/AAP Workshop on Periodontitis and Systemic Diseases. Journal of clinical periodontology 40 Suppl 14:S164-169.

[110] Sembene M, Moreau JC, Mbaye MM, Diallo A, Diallo PD, Ngom M, Benoist HM. 2000. [Periodontal infection in pregnant women and low birth weight babies]. Odontostomatol Trop 23:19-22.

[111] Sharma R, Maimanuku LR, Morse Z, Pack AR. 2007. Preterm low birth weights associated with periodontal disease in the Fiji Islands. International dental journal 57:257-260.

[112] Shetty M, Shetty PK, Ramesh A, Thomas B, Prabhu S, Rao A. 2010. Periodontal disease in pregnancy is a risk factor for preeclampsia. Acta obstetricia et gynecologica Scandinavica 89:718-721.

[113] Siqueira FM, Cota LO, Costa JE, Haddad JP, Lana AM, Costa FO. 2008. Maternal periodontitis as a potential risk variable for preeclampsia: a case-control study. Journal of periodontology 79:207-215.

[114] Skuldbol T, Johansen KH, Dahlen G, Stoltze K, Holmstrup P. 2006. Is pre-term labour associated with periodontitis in a Danish maternity ward? Journal of clinical periodontology 33:177-183.

[115] Soderling E, Isokangas P, Pienihakkinen K, Tenovuo J, Alanen P. 2001. Influence of maternal xylitol consumption on mother-child transmission of mutans streptococci: 6-year follow-up. Caries research 35:173-177.

[116] Srinivas SK, Sammel MD, Stamilio DM, Clothier B, Jeffcoat MK, Parry S, Macones GA, Elovitz MA, Metlay J. 2009. Periodontal disease and adverse pregnancy outcomes: is there an association? American journal of obstetrics and gynecology 200:497 e491-498.

[117] Srivastava A, Gupta KK, Srivastava S, Garg J. 2013. Massive pregnancy gingival enlargement: A rare case. Journal of Indian Society of Periodontology 17:503-506.

[118] Taghzouti N, Xiong X, Gornitsky M, Chandad F, Voyer R, Gagnon G, Leduc L, Xu H, Tulandi T, Wei B, Senecal J, Velly AM, Salah MH, Fraser WD. 2012. Periodontal disease is not associated with preeclampsia in Canadian pregnant women. Journal of periodontology 83:871-877.

[119] Tanner AC, Milgrom PM, Kent R, Jr., Mokeem SA, Page RC, Riedy CA, Weinstein P, Bruss J. 2002. The microbiota of young children from tooth and tongue samples. Journal of dental research 81:53-57.

[120] Tarannum F, Faizuddin M. 2007. Effect of periodontal therapy on pregnancy outcome in women affected by periodontitis. Journal of periodontology 78:2095-2103.

[121] Toygar HU, Seydaoglu G, Kurklu S, Guzeldemir E, Arpak N. 2007. Periodontal health and adverse pregnancy outcome in 3,576 Turkish women. Journal of periodontology 78:2081-2094.

[122] Trindade SC, Gomes-Filho IS, Meyer RJ, Vale VC, Pugliese L, Freire SM. 2008. Serum antibody levels against Porphyromonas gingivalis extract and its chromatographic fraction in chronic and aggressive periodontitis. Journal of the International Academy of Periodontology 10:50-58.

[123] Vergnes JN, Sixou M. 2007. Preterm low birth weight and maternal periodontal status: a meta-analysis. American journal of obstetrics and gynecology 196:135 e131-137.

[124] Verkerk PH, van Noord-Zaadstra BM, Florey CD, de Jonge GA, Verloove-Vanhorick SP. 1993. The effect of moderate maternal alcohol consumption on birth weight and gestational age in a low risk population. Early human development 32:121-129.

[125] Vettore MV, Leal M, Leao AT, da Silva AM, Lamarca GA, Sheiham A. 2008. The relationship between periodontitis and preterm low birthweight. Journal of dental research 87:73-78.

[126] http://en.wikipedia.org/wiki/Vaccine

[127] Wang Y, Sugita N, Kikuchi A, Iwanaga R, Hirano E, Shimada Y, Sasahara J, Tanaka K, Yoshie H. 2012. FcgammaRIIB-nt645+25A/G gene polymorphism and periodontitis in Japanese women with preeclampsia. International journal of immunogenetics 39:492-500.

[128] WHO. 1984. The incidence of low birth weight: an update. World Health Organisation Wkly Epidemiol Rec 59:205-211.

[129] Williams CE, Davenport ES, Sterne JA, Sivapathasundaram V, Fearne JM, Curtis MA. 2000. Mechanisms of risk in preterm low-birthweight infants. Periodontology 2000 23:142-150.

[130] Winkler M, Fischer DC, Hlubek M, van de Leur E, Haubeck HD, Rath W. 1998. Interleukin-1beta and interleukin-8 concentrations in the lower uterine segment during parturition at term. Obstetrics and gynecology 91:945-949.

[131] Wood S, Frydman A, Cox S, Brant R, Needoba S, Eley B, Sauve R. 2006. Periodontal disease and spontaneous preterm birth: a case control study. BMC pregnancy and childbirth 6:24.

[132] Wright HJ, Matthews JB, Chapple IL, Ling-Mountford N, Cooper PR. 2008. Periodontitis associates with a type 1 IFN signature in peripheral blood neutrophils. Journal of immunology 181:5775-5784.

[133] Xiong X, Buekens P, Fraser WD, Beck J, Offenbacher S. 2006. Periodontal disease and adverse pregnancy outcomes: a systematic review. BJOG : an international journal of obstetrics and gynaecology 113:135-143.

[134] Xiong X, Buekens P, Vastardis S, Yu SM. 2007. Periodontal disease and pregnancy outcomes: state-of-the-science. Obstetrical & gynecological survey 62:605-615.

9

Early Childhood Caries (ECC) — Etiology, Clinical Consequences and Prevention

Agim Begzati, Merita Berisha, Shefqet Mrasori, Blerta Xhemajli-Latifi, Rina Prokshi, Fehim Haliti, Valmira Maxhuni, Vala Hysenaj-Hoxha and Vlera Halimi

1. Introduction

Primary teeth are also known as milk or deciduous teeth. The 20 primary teeth start to appear in a baby's mouth around the sixth month and they stay in the mouth until they are gradually replaced by the permanent teeth between the ages of six to twelve years.

Primary teeth start to develop from the 6th to 7th week of fetal life from epithelial cells of the mouth that form the tooth buds. The cells of these initial tooth germs continue to differentiate during pregnancy, and, when the baby is born most teeth are already partially formed in the jaws.

The primary teeth play an important role in giving facial fullness and aesthetically pleasant facial shapes. Absence of teeth, due to any reason, not only hampers the masticatory activity of the individual, but also affect the facial features to great extent, affecting the concerned person physiologically, emotionally and socially.

Unfortunately, the primary teeth's function is disrupted when the demineralization process of hard tooth structures is involved – dental caries.

The oral health of children is especially aggravated with the occurrence of the so-called early childhood caries(ECC). ECC is an acute, rapidly developing dental disease occurring initially in the cervical third of the maxillary incisors, destroying the crown completely.

The presence of dental caries, especially of ECC, may reflect on the oral health status of children in countries with insufficient health system and inefficient primary dentistry. Early Childhood Caries (ECC) is a public health problem with biological, social and behavioral determinants.

The preventive activities must start at an early age. Home-care methods are more than necessary.

1.1. Primary Teeth

The eruption of the primary teeth starts around the sixth month with the central incisors of the lower jaw and it is fully completed by the 3rd year of age with the appearance of the upper second molar. Normally, the first teeth that erupt are the two front teeth of the lower jaw (mandibular central incisors). After a few of months they are followed by the four front teeth of the upper jaw (maxillary central and lateral incisors). The last primary teeth that erupt are the upper second molars which are expected to appear around the age of 2½ years and not later than the completion of the 3rd year.

Teeth eruption is the process during which they move towards the surface of the jawbone and break through the gums, until they take their final position in the mouth with their crown fully visible. At this point the crown is completely formed, but the root of the tooth will continue to form for one more year.

The process of tooth eruption is usually accompanied with pain and discomfort for the baby. The associated symptoms such as drooling, disruptions in eating or sleeping patterns, irritability, swollen gums are referred as 'teething'.

When the primary dentition is completed, children have a set of 20 primary teeth, ten at every jaw. They belong to 3 different teeth types: 8 incisors, 4 canines, and 8 molars.

Eruption of the first permanent molar (age of 6 years), marks the end of the primary dentition period and the start of mixed dentition.

The anatomy and morphology of the primary teeth is also generally similar with that of permanent teeth. Externally the tooth is covered by a layer of enamel at the crown area and by cementum at the root area. Under the enamel there is a layer of dentine which surrounds the soft and alive dental pulp at the center of the tooth.

However some distinctive features of primary teeth are: smaller size, thinner and more translucent enamel, less mineralized enamel (which makes primary teeth more vulnerable to cavities, especially for early childhood caries), larger pulp chambers, narrower and smaller roots, etc.

1.2. Role/importance of the primary teeth

Parents commonly ask why they should worry about cavities in baby, since they will be replaced by the permanent teeth? The role of the primary teeth is just as important as the role of the permanent ones.

Humans use teeth to tear, grind, and chew food in the first step of digestion. Teeth also play a role in human speech. Additionally, teeth also provide structural support to muscles in the face and form the human smile and other facial expressions. So, broadly the main functions of the teeth can be summarized as follows: role in mastication (helps eating), aids in articulation and speech, role in aesthetics (gives shape and beauty to the face).

One of the main functions of teeth is the mastication of the food. The first step of digestion involves the mouth and teeth. Each type of tooth serves a different function in the chewing process. Depending on the shape, teeth enable cutting, grinding, chewing and preparing food for swallow and further digestion in the digestive tract. The Incisors cut foods when you bite into them. The sharper and longer canines tear food, while the wider molars grind the food.

Masticatory function, besides stimulating the development of the jaws, allows the child to learn the right way of eating. Toothache during mastication can affect the child's nutrition. According to some studies it has been found that children with more decayed teeth have less than 80% of average weight, which they are expected to have for their age (Acs et al 1999, Acs et al 1992). Children with toothache often after their recovery reach their normal weight and have tranquility during their sleep (Elice & Fields 1990).

The role of healthy primary teeth consists in clearly speaking and emphasizing the correct letters and sounds. The mouth, especially the teeth, lips, and tongue are essential for speech, one of the very important functions of teeth. The teeth, lips, and tongue are used to form words by controlling airflow through the mouth. Especially, the front teeth enable correct pronunciation of consonants: t, th, d, f, etc.

Primary teeth, among other roles, have one more extremely important role. As long as they are in the oral cavity, until their physiological loss, they will serve as space retention for permanent teeth. Their premature loss can be a cause of malocclusions in children. If we achieve to prevent their premature loss, malocclusion frequency will be reduced for 30%. Although early loss of primary incisors would not have a major consequence, a premature loss of primary molar and canine will be marked by a significant disorder in the development of occlusion during the eruption of the permanent teeth (Marković 1976).

Healthy teeth and full realization of their function, in fact, will allow a normal psycho-physical development of children, which for their age, is very important.

2. Dental caries — Definition, etiology and epidemiology

Dental caries is one of the most prevalent diseases in children worldwide. The Center for Disease Control and Prevention reports that dental caries is perhaps the most prevalent infectious diseases in children. Dental caries is five times more common than asthma and seven times more common than hay fever in children (US Department of Health and Human Services 2000).

Tooth decay is localized progressive disease, whose character consists in the destruction of tooth structures mainly under the influence of metabolic products of the oral microflora.

Dental caries is pathological destruction of tooth hard tissue with progressive effluence. Initially it appears in enamel, the dentin is involved after that, and later the pulp and the periodontium, with the possibility of complications that will affect the general health. The consequences of caries may be numerous, ranging from the morphological changes to functional ones, e.g. complete crown destruction (early childhood caries), chewing difficulties, speech impediments, digestive tract disorders, odentogenic focal points (Raiç 1985, Stosic 1991).

Dental caries usually begins as small, shallow holes; if left untreated, these holes can become larger and deeper and potentially lead to tooth destruction or loss. Complications of dental caries include: pain, dental abscess, difficulties during chewing, tooth damage or loss, tooth sensitivity.

There are numerous definitions on caries, depending on what is taken in consideration: etiology, pathogenesis, clinical features.

Dental caries may be defined as a bacterial disease of the hard tissues of the teeth characterized by demineralization of the inorganic and destruction of the organic substance of tooth (Soames & Southam 1999).

According to Douglas, dental caries is the most common chronic infectious disease of childhood, caused by the interaction of bacteria, mainly *Streptococcus mutans*, and sugary foods on tooth enamel. *S. mutans* breaks down sugars for energy, causing an acidic environment in the mouth and result in demineralization of the enamel of the teeth and dental caries (Douglass et al. 2004).

Since *S. mutans* is transmitted to the child, another definition is based in the transmissibility. Dental caries is defined as a transmissible localized infection caused by a multi-factorial etiology. In order for dental caries to develop, four interrelated factors must occur: the patient (host), substrate (carbohydrates), dental plaque (*S. mutans*), and the time factor.

2.1. Etiology

Dental caries is a disease that is not caused by one factor. If only one factor would cause this disease, its prevention would have been much easier and more controllable. Many studies like clinical studies, but mostly longitudinal epidemiological studies, show convincing evidence for a multi-factorial nature of this disease. Numerous factors affecting the appearance of caries act team-wise and not separately, make caries pathogenesis very complex but also hinder the possibility to undertake effective preventive measures.

There are several important factors that make up the dental caries etiological circle. Host respectively tooth, dental plaque respectively bacteria, and substrate respectively saliva carbohydrates, all in co-operation with the time factor, are vicious chain of dental caries development.

The hard tooth structure, the enamel, is the forefront part that undergoes the demineralization process, respectively caries. The development of caries in enamel surface as much as it is affected by the internal structure of the hard tissue build of the tooth, equally, perhaps even more it depends on the strength of external factors affect.

Sometimes for various reasons: local, general or even hereditary, tooth structure can be so poorly mineralized, that it would need a very small amount of external factors to cause dental caries.

The general opinion regarding the etiology of dental caries nowadays is that it is a very complex multifactorial disease, presented with high prevalence in all age groups. It has already been established that dental caries is a chronic infectious process with a multifactorial etiology. Dietary factors, oral microorganisms that can produce acids from sugars, and host suscepti- bility all need to coexist for caries to develop (Konig & Navia 1995).

There are some important factors that comprise the etiological circles of the dental caries: host or the tooth, dental or bacterial plaque, substrate – carbohydrates and saliva, and altogether co-react with the time factor. The hard dental structures, initially the enamel, undergo the demineralization process, respectively the caries. The caries development in the enamel surface is equally dependent from the inner hard dental structure and from the intensity of the extrinsic factors' action.

The newest concept in dentistry explains the cause of dental caries as a consequence of disruption of "Caries Balance" (Featherstone 2004). Dr. John Featherstone introduced the concept of the Caries Balance in 2002. The theory of "Caries Balance" defines dental caries as a disease of hard dental tissues, and the destruction of the enamel surface as a result of the disruption of the balance of demineralization and remineralization.

This misbalance may be manifested in the beginning of demineralization or during the process of remineralization. The defect in the enamel surface is a result of the domination of the demineralization process and such process has progressive course directed towards pulpar space. Which process will dominate depends on the proportions of the factors that constitute "Caries Balance", i.e. protective and pathological factors.

The balance disorder will be manifested with early demineralization process or eventually with remineralization process. This concept is that dental caries can be viewed as a balance of healthy or protective factors (factor of remineralization), and disease or pathogenic factors (factor of demineralization). Cavities are caused by an imbalance between risk factors for the disease and protective factors.

Pathological factors (risk factors) are: acid-producing bacteria, frequent eating/drinking of fermentable carbohydrates, sub-normal saliva flow and "function".

Protective factors are: saliva flow and its components; fluoride, calcium, phosphate reminer- alization; antibacterials (chlorhexidine, xylitol), etc.

The level of risk for dental caries depends on the domination of the certain group of factors that participate in the "Caries Balance". If there is domination of the pathological factors, the risk for dental caries will be higher and the treatment needs will require larger restorative interventions, as well as other consequences. If there is a domination of protective factors, then the invasive restorative dentistry will have fewer burdens, and concentrate in minimal restorations of superficial caries. Biological factors tend to be similar within all cultures and populations, although habit/environmental factors tend to be influenced specifically by the culture in place.

2.2. The prevalence of dental caries

It has already been mentioned that dental caries is the mostly spread disease in the world. Dental caries is a disease that affects all age groups, most commonly children.

Epidemiological data derived from the Oral Health Promotion Group of Kosovo showed a high prevalence of caries among children in Kosovo (89.2% among preschool children and 94.4% among school children). The mean dmft/DMFT index was 5.6 for preschool children and 4.9 for all school children (Begzati et al. 2011).

The results from the same previous study show that dental health of these children in Kosovo is worse than that of children in other European countries. Specifically, the mean dmft of five-year-olds at preschools in Kosovo (8.1) was found to be higher than the same value of preschool children in USA (1.7) and in many other European countries (1991-1995), including Ireland (0.9), Spain (1.0), Denmark (1.3), Norway (1.4), Finland (1.4), Netherlands (1.7), United Kingdom (2.0), France (2.5), and Germany (2.5). Our results are only comparable to the rates in Belarus (7.4), Sarajevo, Bosnia (7.53) (ages 5-7) and Albania (8.5), (Marthaler 1996, Kobaslia 2000). The low treatment rate of children in Kosovo (<2%) indicates a high treatment need. Also, the mean DMFT (5.8) of school children in Kosovo (age 12) was higher in comparison with school children (age 12) of the following developed countries: Netherlands (1.1), Finland (1.2), Denmark (1.3), USA (1.4), United Kingdom (1.4), Sweden (1.5), Norway (2.1), Ireland (2.1), Germany (2.6) and Croatia (2.6) (16). The mean DMFT of Kosovo's children (age 12) was similar to the mean values in Latvia (7.7), Poland (5.1) and a group of 12- to 14-year-olds in Sarajevo, Bosnia (7.18), (Marthaler 1996, Kobaslia 2000).

3. Early Childhood Caries (ECC)-definition

ECC is an acute, rapidly developing dental disease occurring initially in the cervical third of the maxillary incisors, destroying the crown completely. Early onset and rampant clinical progression makes ECC a serious public health problem. Due to varying clinical, etiological,

localization, and course features, this pathology is found under different names such as labial caries (LC), caries of incisors, nursing bottle mouth, rampant caries (RC), nursing bottle caries (NBC), nursing caries, baby bottle tooth decay (BBTD), early childhood caries (ECC), rampant early childhood dental decay, and severe early childhood caries (SECC) (James 1957, Goose 1967, Fass 1962, Winter et al.1966, Derkson & Ponti 1982, Ripa 1988, Arkin 1986, Bruered et al. 1989, Kaste & Gift 1995, Tinanoff et al. 1998, Horowitz 1998, Drury et al. 1999).

According to Davis, the definition of this pathology has always been complex and "difficult to be described, but when it is seen, you know what it's about" (Davis 1998).

In 1862, an American physician, Abraham Jacobi (Jacobi 1862) was the first to describe the clinical appearance of early childhood caries, which he observed in one of his own patients. Whereas, in 1932 Beltrami described this form of caries, as "Les dentes noires des tout petits" (black teeth in small children), (Beltrami 1952). Author Fass, created the term *nursing bottle mouth* (Fass 1962).

The literature contains a variety of other terms used to describe early childhood caries and its diagnostic criteria. Most of them relate to the use of a feeding bottle or prolonged breastfeeding (feeding bottle tooth decay, feeding bottle syndrome, nursing caries, nursing bottle mouth, and so on). The authors wish to highlight the danger of excessive drinking from a baby bottle, if it contains sweetened liquids, or prolonged on-demand breastfeeding (Schroth et al. 2007).

To inform the scientific community with internationally comparable data on the incidence of early childhood caries, delegates to a conference at the Centers for Disease Control and Prevention, invented the term *early childhood caries* in order to better the multi-factorial pathogenesis of the disease" (Kaste & Gift 1995).

Unfortunately, this term was seen to have its limitations. Three years later, a further conference on early childhood caries, organized by the National Health Institute (USA), added two further definitions/descriptions, which were *rampant infant caries* and *early childhood dental decay* (RIE, CDD), (Quartey & Williamson 1998). These differences in definition were due above all to diversity in diagnostic criteria.

3.1. Clinical diagnostic criteria of Early Childhood Caries (ECC)

Due to the early appearance, typical localization, rapid destruction of the hard tissue of tooth, early childhood caries is a specific form of primary tooth decay. Childhood caries appears in caries resistant regions, such as: labial surfaces of the upper incisors, in the upper and lower molars, more rarely in the upper canine, and even less or not at all in the lower canine and incisors. In addition, during bottle-feeding with sugar-containing drinks, the upper incisors bathe in these sugar-containing drinks but the saliva from minor salivary glands in the area of these teeth has only limited remineralising properties, whereas the lower incisors remain largely protected by the tongue during bottle-feeding.

Different authors propose different criteria to define or describe the early childhood caries. Author Amidi, studying the publications about ECC, has concluded that: in 27 publications, the criteria for defining ECC was the presence of labial surface caries in at least one frontal maxillary tooth, in 23 studies at least two frontal maxillary teeth while in 9 studies three frontal maxillary teeth (Soames & Southam 1999).

Below are some criteria's for defining early childhood caries from various researchers cited by authors Amid & Woosung 1999:

- involvement of one or more maxillary incisors, without the involvement of mandibular incisors- author Sewint;

- a white or black spot in the labial surface of the maxillary frontal teeth- author Bennitz;

- one or more carious lesions in maxillary incisors, along gingival margin- author Ayhan;

- carious lesions in labial-buccal surfaces at one or more maxillar incisors- author Ramos;

- two or more maxillar incisors- author Harrison.

In the literature we still can find some criteria's, for example:

- one or more frontal maxillary teeth that has evidence that the child was fed with a bottle (Al-Dashti 1995);

- maxillar incisors and the mesial surface of canine (O'Sallivan 1993);

- at least one carious maxillary incisor with the involvement of labial and proximal surface or only proximale surface (Kaste et al. 1996);

- one or more maxillary incisor with cervical crown caries (Lopez 1998).

Author Wynne 1999, classifies early childhood caries into three types:

Type I (moderately easy) - usually involves two upper central incisors.

Type II (moderate, severe) - includes incisors, first molar, canine, and does not include the lower incisors.

Type III (widespread, severe) - including the mandibular incisors.

3.2. ECC — Prevalence

Prevalence of ECC is different and it largely depends on the criteria set by the researcher and the place where the examination takes place. There are differences between the data for urban or rural places, rich or poor places, "flourished" or "non-flourished" places. Furthermore, the prevalence of ECC varies in different countries, which may depend on the diagnostic criteria. While in some developed countries having advanced programs for oral health protection, the prevalence of ECC is around 5% (Derkson & Ponti 1982, Ripa 1988, Kaste et al. 1996, Davenport 1990, Hinds & Gregory 1995). In some countries of Southeastern Europe (neighboring countries of Kosovo) this prevalence reaches 20% (Bosnia) and 14% (Macedonia) (Huseinbegović 2001, Apostolova et al. 2003). Much higher ECC prevalence has been reported for such places as Quchan, Iran (59%) (Mazhari et al. 2007) and Alaska (66.8%) (Kelly & Bruerd 1987). At American Indian children the prevalence is 41.8% (Kelly & Bruerd 1987). Similarly, in North American populations, the prevalence at high-risk children ranges from 11% to 72% (Berkowitz 2003).

Data from relevant literature show different prevalence in different countries, cited by various authors (Berkowitz et al. 1993, McDonald 2000, Wendet 1995, Begzati et al. 2011, Barbakov et al. 1985, Harris & Garsia 1999, Huseinbegović 2001, Holt et al. 1996, Kaste 1991, Pettit et al. 2001, Bruered et al.1989, Reisine 1998, Wyne 1999, Apostolova 2003).

3.3. Etiology

Dental caries is an infectious and transmissible disease. Therefore, early childhood caries is an extremely aggressive form of the disease.

It was suggested that from the biological determinants, the three key causal factors for dental caries were: microorganisms, substrate, and host (Keyes 1962).

However, in the etiology of early childhood caries very special role given to dental plaque, respectively cariogenic bacteria. Of the great interest in the cariogenesis process are only two

Place (year)	Author	Age	Prevalence
England(1989)	Silver	3 years	4%
Sweden1991)	Wendet	12-14 months	4.7%
Finland (1993)	Paunio	3 years	6%
Irak (1990)	Yagoot	1-5 years	15.6%
Kosova (2011)	Begzati	2-6 y.	17.5%
Indonesia (1979)	Aldy, Siregar	Up to 5 years	48%
Bosnia (2001)	Huseinbegović	5 y.	29%
Nigeria (1985)	Salako	3-7 y.	38.4%
Canada (1987)	Budowski	1-5 y.	7.4%
USA (1976)	Kaste	One years	0.8-2%
USA(1991)	Kaste	5 y.	5%
USA (1991)	Kamp	4 y.	5.3%
USA (1987)	Brured	3-5y.,native Indians Amer., and Alaska's population,	41.8-66.8%
USA (1992)	Weinstetin,	Mexican American, 8-47 m.	29.6%
Italia (2002)	Petti, Iannazzo	3-5 y.	7.6%
Macedonia (2003)	Apostolova	3 y.	13.3%
Australia (1998)	Reisine	Aborigin children	50%
Saudi Arabia	Wynne	Preschool children	15%
Kuwait (1986)	Soparkar	4-5 y.	11.5%

bacterial genera: mutant streptococci and lactobacills (Norman & Franklin 1999). A very important role is attributed to the bacterium Streptococcus mutans-called "the window of infection" (Caufield et al. 1993), in that it is responsible for the primary oral infection in the first phase of ECC (Berkowitz 1980; Berkowitz et al. 1996).

The most important requirement is an early infection, usually with the mother's cariogenic bacteria, for example, between the age of 19-31 months. However, earlier and later infection is a possibility (Caufield et al. 1993, Wan 2001).

After transmission of cariogenic bacteria and a frequent supply of substrate (sucrose) to the plaque, usually given as a sugary drink (juices and so on from a feeding bottle) or in older children, in snacks in the form of solid-cariogenic foods such as sweets, chocolates, cakes, biscuits, the development of early childhood caries occurs. If this loading of the plaque with sugars occurs at bedtime (night) and there is no tooth brushing, caries can progress rapidly.

In addition to the other severe types of early childhood caries, feeding on demand with cariogenic food and liquids is regarded as a co-factor for early childhood caries (Wendt & Birkhed 1995). As mentioned earlier, many social and behavioral determinants are risk factors for early childhood caries.

Favoring risk factors are as follows: low socio-economic status, low educational attainment in parents, chronic non-communicable diseases, inadequate health literacy, are all risk factors for a early childhood caries. Social and behavioral factors have been described in association with early childhood caries in numerous publications (FDI 1988, Horowitz 1998, Reisine & Douglass 1998, Seow 1998).

3.3.1. Cariogenic bacteria

In one of our studies conducted in the clinic of Paediatric Dentistry, it was found that S.mutans had a crucial role in ECC. The prevalence of S.mutans at our children was around 90% (Begzati et al. 2014). These facultative anaerobes are commonly found in the human oral cavity, and are a major contributor of tooth decay. The result of decay can greatly affect the overall health of the individual (Whiley & Beighton 2013).

The mutans streptococci and some Lactobacillus species are the two groups of infectious agents most strongly associated with dental caries. Earlier clinical studies reported that MS could not be detected in the mouths of normal predentate infants (Berkowitz et al. 1975, Berkowitz et al. 1980, Stiles et al. 1976, Catalanotto et al. 1975, Caufield et al. 1993, Karn et al 1998).

More recent clinical investigations have demonstrated that MS can colonize in the mouths of predentate infants (Tanner et al. 2002; Wan et al. 2001).

According to Berkowitz transmission of S.mutans happens in two ways: vertical and horizontal transmission. Vertical transmission is the transmission of microbes from caregiver to child. The major reservoir from which infants acquire S.mutans is their mothers. A study conducted by Berkowitz and co-authors reported that, when mothers harbored greater than 10^5 colony forming units (cfu) of MS per mL of saliva, the frequency of infant infection was 58%. When mothers harbored 10^3 cfu of MS per mL of saliva or more, however, the frequency of infant infection was 9 times less (6%) (Berkowitz et al 1981). These data clearly demonstrate that mothers with dense salivary reservoirs of MS are at high risk for infecting their infants early in life.

Vertical transmission is not the only vector by which MS are perpetuated in human populations.

Horizontal transmission also occurs. Horizontal transmission is the transmission of microbes between members of a group (eg, family members of a similar age or students in a classroom). Based on appearance, ways of transmission and prevention, Berkowitz concludes that: primary oral infection by mutans streptococci (MS) may occur in predentate infants. Infants may acquire MS via vertical and horizontal transmission. Improvements in the prevention of dental caries may likely be realized through intervention strategies that focus on the natural history of this infectious disease.

Streptococcus mutans (SM)

Streptococcus mutans are gram-positive cocci shaped bacteria. SM is isolated from all tissues of the oral cavity and constitutes the largest number of inhabitants of the oral microflora. This bacteria belongs to the Viridans group of streptococci (Galdvin 2004). Traditionally oral streptococci are differentiated on the basis of simple biochemical and physiological tests. Many recent studies comparing homologous DNA, gave description of the whole protein content and detection of glicosidasis activity clarifying the relationship between many species.

Mutant streptococci represent a group of bacterial species that had previously been classified as serotypes of the same species. These bacteria are characterized by their ability to ferment manitol and sorbitol, producing extracellular glicanes from sucrose with cariogenic activity in animal models. Important for the human population are two species: S. mutans and S. sobrinus. Streptococcus mutans has got this name in 1924 when Clarke in England isolated the microorganisms from human carious lesions. He noted that they are more oval shaped, not round and assumed that they are mutants of streptococcus.

Mutant streptococci, are now considered as the main pathogenic species involved in the caries process. It is noted that if they are seeded in the mouth of animals, including rats, rodents and monkeys, are able to cause caries. Some detailed studies have shown a correlation between the presence of S.mutans and caries. These findings are repeated in longitudinal studies of microbiology and caries incidence. Mutant streptococci are usually found in relatively large numbers in plaque formed immediately after the development of lesions at the superficial soft surfaces. During a longitudinal study samples are taken periodically for analysis of separate parts for S.mutans and teeth were examined simultaneously. Teeth destined to become decayed, showed a significant increase of the ratio of S.mutans 6 to 24 months before the eventual diagnosis of caries. In similar conditions SM isolated from dental plaque terrains on stained white lesions are characterized by a ratio greater than plaque by SM while probing enamel grounds. The increased number of SM in saliva has also gone hand in hand with the development of lesions in smooth surface. In another study of saliva analysis of 200 children showed that 93 percent of them were positive for caries evident S. mutant, while uninfected children were almost always unaffected by decay (Russell 2003).

S. mutans position as the primary agent of caries formation in favor of their certain physiological characteristics. These features include the ability to adhere in tooth surface, producing insoluble polysaccharides from sucrose, rapidly producing lactic acid substrates by a number of sugars, acid tolerance and formation of intracellular stores of polysaccharides. These features help cariogenic SM survival in an environment not suitable in terms of so-called "feast or famine" cycles or due to the low concentration of substrate (i.e between meals) or excess substrate concentrations (e.g during consumption of food rich in sugar). As a general rule, cariogenic bacteria metabolize sugars to produce energy they need for growth and multiplication. The products of this metabolism are acids, which are derived from bacteria in plaque fluid. Damage caused by S.mutans is mainly due to lactic acid, although other acids such as butyric and propionic was found within the plaque. Generally, S.mutans is the most common streptococcal mutant infectious agent in humans and strong evidences are presented as the most virulent cause of odontogenic infections. Another mutans bacteria from the group of so-called S.sobrinus, differs from S.mutans because they require sucrose for adherence and growth in the dental plaque.

Correlation between caries and S. mutans, based on the data described in the literature and based on experimental models that are performed, and based on certain conclusions (Russell 2003):

- Animal experiments: S. mutans causes caries among gnatobiotik animals in the presence of sugar;

- Virulence: S. mutans has properties that contribute to caries development. These properties are acidogenety, uric acid production, extarcelular production of glicanes and intracellular storage of polysaccharides;

- Cross-sectional studies in humans: an increase in the number of S. mutans found in the initial carious lesions;

- Longitudinal studies in humans: a large number of S. mutans in a number of tooth decays correlates with subsequent caries;

- Streptococci other "non mutans" with similar properties can also be cariogenic.

S.mutans, sugar and caries

Taking large amounts of sugar combined with low values of pH frequently leads to an increased number of S. mutans.These bacteria are characterized by these features:

- Capacity to adhere to tooth structure

- Sugar Transportation system

- Production of lactic acid from sugars

- Production of intra and extracellular polysaccharide

- Tolerance in acidic environment

S. mutans sugar transportation

S. mutans is equipped with a conveyor system more efficient to carry sugars within their cells. During the metabolic process in the cell, they produce different substances, which contribute sufficiently to their pathogenicity. When it received the greatest amount of sugars S. mutans produce mainly Lactic Acid (Hamada and Slade, 1980). Streptococcus mutans produces extracellular and intracellular polysaccharides. Extracellular polysaccharides are also produced during the enzymatic reactions. Their sticky properties are favorable for bacterial adherence capabilities on the surface of the teeth, helping their placement on smooth surfaces (Koga 1986, Loesch 1986).

Polysaccharides also help connectivity and multiplication of dental plaque. Moreover, their insolubility prevents natural protective effect of saliva. Polysaccharides ensure the survival of intracellular bacteria in nutritionally poor intervals, and are used by bacteria to produce acids (Hamada and Slade 1980).

S. mutans, tolerance to acidic environment

Bacteria multiply under certain environmental conditions and they have obvious advantages compared with other micro-organisms. Diet and lack of suppressive factors determine the composition of the oral flora.

The decrease in pH prevents many bacteria from growth, while streptococci are multiplying in this particular environment (Harper & Loesch 1984). Changes in bacterial flora are in favor of bacteria which can survive in acidic conditions on account of acid no-tolerant microorganisms and acidic production. Pathogenic micro-organisms produce acid, the pH of which is lower enough than the value below which the tooth enamel begins to melt. S. mutans is recognized as the initiator of caries. They affect the initiation of the process leading to loss of minerals, and this facilitates the bacteria to penetrate the tooth structure (Burne 1998).

3.3.2. Substrate (Carbohydrates)

The human body uses glucose as substrate food, while other carbohydrates under the action of relevant enzymes converted into glucose. Cariotic action of sugars depends on their fermenting potential, respectively as far as the highest level of acids produced by the their fermentation. It was found that carbohydrates are the major class fermentabile affecting ecological changes in the mouth. While carbohydrates are transformed into acids, sucrose under the action of bacterial enzymes (glykosiltransferasa-GTF, and fruktosyltransferasa-FTF) turns into two classes polymers (glukan and fruktan).

Glukan plays the role of infectious matter to the surface of the tooth, not dissolved in water. This attribute enables attachment of dental plaque and S.mutans for tooth surface. Levan under the influence of enzymes derived from S. mutans fermented in the acidic product (Pincaham 1994).

Dairy products (milk, cheese) has an influence in the ecology of the area of the mouth. Dairy products can protect teeth from decay. This can happen as a result of buffer capacity of milk proteins or because of decarboxylation of amino acids after proteolysis some bacteria can metabolise kazein. Milk protein (casein) and its derivatives can be absorbed on the surface of the tooth, modify the structure of pelicula which make it unsuitable for adhesion of S. mutans, but also enable establishing of calcium phosphate and initiate the process of remineralisation.

Some sugar substitutes that do not turn into acid, as xilitoli for example you add sweets, have a role in inhibiting the development of S. Mutans (Pincaham 1994, Marsh 2000).

Correlation between SM and consumption of sugars

Studies on the correlation between presence of SM in saliva and sweet diet is not entirely clear, even data from the literature are sometimes contradictory. While some studies such as those of Polish authors has shown that children with a SM presence is 94% while 56% LB and daily frequency of sweets consumption exceeds 5 times a day (Wierzbicka, 1987). But, so it does not happen with children in Mozambique where annual consumption of sugar for school children is very low (11 kg), while the presence of SM is 98%, 40% of their high value. Sudan is also similar in that although annual consumption is about 18 kg, SM was identified in 90%, moderate values and higher than 50% (Carlsson 1989).

4. Study report

In our previous study (Begzati et al. 2010), the prevalence of ECC and various caries risk factors such as quantity of cariogenic S mutans colonies, was evaluated.

Methods

In the study there were included 1,008 children of both sexes, from 1 to 6 years of age, from 9 kindergartens of Prishtina, capital city of Kosovo. The sample was random, representing 80% of all kindergarten children. The sample size was calculated with a confidence level of 95% and a confidence interval of 2.

Bacterial sampling — Determination of S.mutans

In our study the presence of S mutans was determined using the CRT bacteria test (Ivoclar Vivadent, Liechtenstein) on the saliva previously stimulated by chewing paraffin. Bacterial counts were recorded as colony-forming units per milliliter (CFU/mL) of saliva. The number of bacterial colonies was graded as follows: Class 0 and Class 1 (CFU < 105/mL saliva), and Class 2 and Class 3 (CFU ≥ 105/mL saliva), according to the manufacturers' scoring-card (Ivoclar-Vivadent, Lichtenstein). In younger subjects, with less saliva collected, the modified spatula method was used.

Dental examination and diagnostic criteria

The children were examined in well-lit premises, using a flashlight as the light source, and a dental mirror and dental probe. Diagnostic criteria were calibrated (Hunt 1986), with inter-examiner reliability resulting in kappa = 0.91, based on the examination of 35 children of different ages. Dental caries was scored as the number of decayed, missing, or filled primary teeth (dmft).

ECC was defined as "initial occurrence of caries in cervical region of at least two maxillary incisors." Using a careful lift-the-lip examination, the presence or absence of ECC was recorded depending on the presence of "noncavity caries/white spot lesions" or "cavity caries."

In order to study the clinical and etiological aspects of ECC, a sub-sample of children with ECC was included for further analysis. The latter part of the examination, which included the clinical study of ECC development (according to ECC stages), determination of bacterial colony sampling, oral hygiene index (OHI), and filling out of the questionnaire, was conducted in the Pediatric Dentistry Clinic of the School of Dentistry.Children with ECC were examined using the light of the dental unit, with dental mirror and probe.

Clinical course of ECC

In order to explain the clinical course of ECC, we propose the following stages in the occurrence and progression of carious lesions in ECC: ECCi (initial stage), ECCc (circular stage), ECC_d (destructive stage) and ECC_r (*radix relicta* stage).

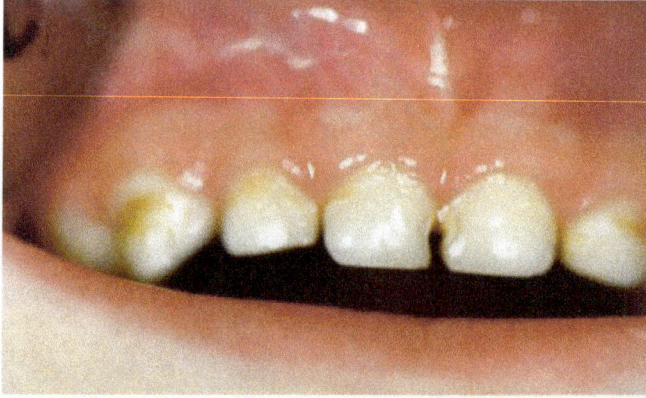

Figure 1. ECCi (initial stage)—white spot lesion or initial defect in enamel of cervix.

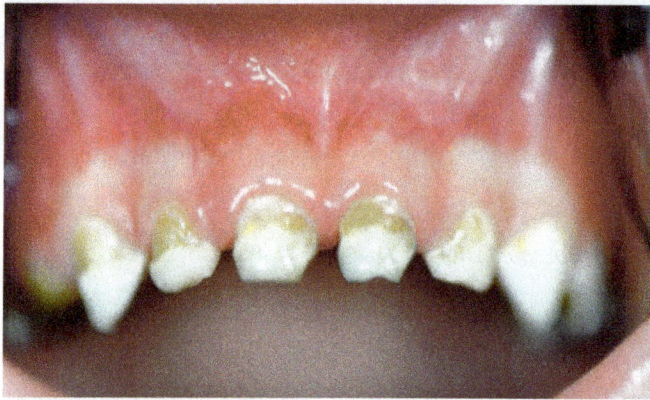

Figure 2. ECCc (circular stage)—lesion in the dentin and circular distribution of this lesion proximally.

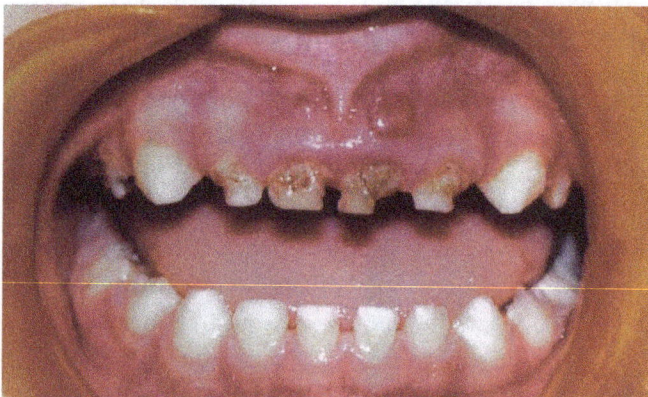

Figure 3. ECC_d (destructive stage)—destruction of more than half the crown without affecting the incisal edge.

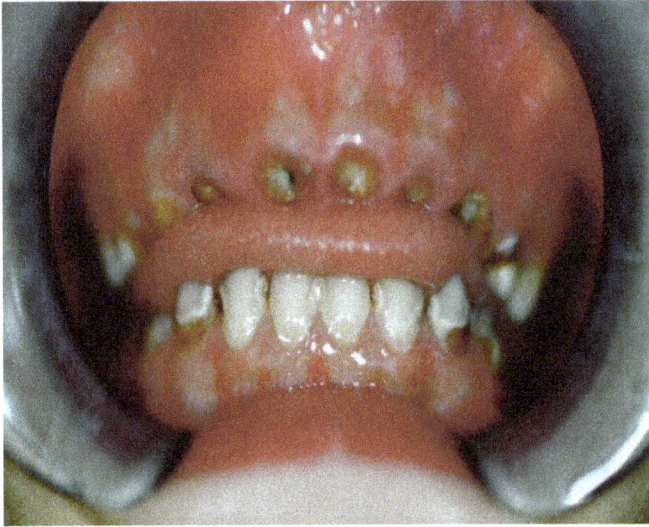

Figure 4. ECC, (*radix relicta* stage) — total destruction of the crown.

Results of study

From the total 1,008 examined children aged 1-6 years, the caries prevalence expressed in terms of the caries index per person, or dmft > 0, was 86.31%, with a mean dmft of 5.8. The prevalence of ECC was 17.36%, or 175 out of 1,008 examined children (Figure 1). The sub-sample of children with diagnosed ECC consisted of 150 children out of 175 invited for further analysis. Twentyfive children of this group from different kindergartens didn't show up in the Department. The mean age of children with ECC was 3.8 ± 1.2 years. The mean dmft in children with ECC was 11 ± 3.6. There was no statistical difference of ECC prevalence between genders (t test = 1.81, P = 0.07).

As expected, the lowest mean dmft score was found at age 2 (6.47 ± 2.13), with an age-related increase in dmft of 12.8 at age 6 (Table 1). In comparing the mean dmft in ECC children with respect to age, there was a significant statistical difference between age 2 and ages 4, 5, and 6. (One-Way ANOVA test F = 16, P < 0.001).

ECC stages

The ECC stages were not equally distributed. The most common stage present was that of radix relicta (41.7%), while the stage appearing least frequently was the initial stage (15.4%), or 27 out of 150 children with ECC.

There was a significant difference between the stages of ECC (c2 = 211.1, P < 0.0001). Twenty-five of the 27 children with ECC in the initial stage were reexamined 1 year after the baseline examination (2 children did not appear for reexamination dueto address change). The 1-year reexamination showed that the initial stage had advanced to the circular stage in 28% of cases, destructive stage in 20%, radix relicta stage in 36%, and having been extracted due to ECC in 16% of cases (Table 2). Mean age of subjects with initial stage of ECC was 2 ± 0.7. Mean dmft on reexamination showed an increase from 5.1 to 8.8 (P < 0.001).

4.1. Clinical specificities and progress

Even before the child is 2 years, in the gingival third of the labial surface of the upper front teeth, as a result of the enamel decalcification process a chalk colored stain ("white spot lesions") appears, which expands in the enamel of the cervical region of the tooth and for a short time it covers the entire tooth, destroying the whole hard tooth tissue. During this process, initially the enamel on the incisal region of the frontal tooth is resistant, especially canine, that shows that those parts of tooth enamel which are mineralized before birth, are more resistant to caries than the parts that are mineralized after birth (Thomas et al. 1999).

In the initial stage(Fig.1) there is a small loss of minerals from the hydroxylapatite crystals of enamel. As a result of tooth's hard tissue demineralization micropores start forming, which refract the light, and as a result it comes to the formation of so-called *white spots lesions*. Such spots are localized where the concentration of dental plaque is higher. If the destruction continues as a result of the demineralization effect of acids on enamel and apatite removal, the cavity starts to form. (Reisine & Douglass 1998).

This quick progress, helps the caries to quickly affect even the dentin layer, so for a short time the entire tooth crown is destroyed and all that remain are the roots (radix relicta)(Fig.4). Often it happens in 3 year old children, in the upper frontal region, where they have only roots remaining that resemble stumps.

Iritative formation of dentin, which makes the carious lesion get a brown color is a result of permanent irritation in the revealed dentin, while sclerotic tissue can make a full obliteration of tooth canal. The formation of iritative – sclerotic dentin can have an effect in this disease without symptoms, but with difficulties in feeding, speech and aesthetics. Also as a result of reflexive reaction (gums, tongue, lips injury etc.), a number of general symptoms is provoked such as digestive disorders, raised body temperature, increased saliva production, etc. The dental pain starts when the tooth pulp is revealed, in gangrenous teeth or when the infectious pathological process appears in periodoncium.

4.2. Complications and consequences

Early crown destruction – root remaining (radix relicta)

Sometimes, in the upper fornix we can see several changes that, in a quick glance, can lead us to the wrong diagnosis. Since the permanent teeth have palatine position, during their eruption process they put internal pressure in the apical part of the deciduous teeth, so that the deciduous tooth root tip can penetrate the bone and mucosa and erupt in the upper level of vestibular fornix (Fig.5). The erupted roots can make deep and painful decubitus at the upper lip (Fig. 8)

If in the root canal a purulent or gangrenous inflammatory process is present, then in the upper fornix we may encounter isolated purulent process (encapsulated) - abscess. (Fig. 6)

Extension of the inflammatory process - sometimes purulent inflammatory process involves gingiva, on all remaining roots, where the clinical symptoms become much more difficult.

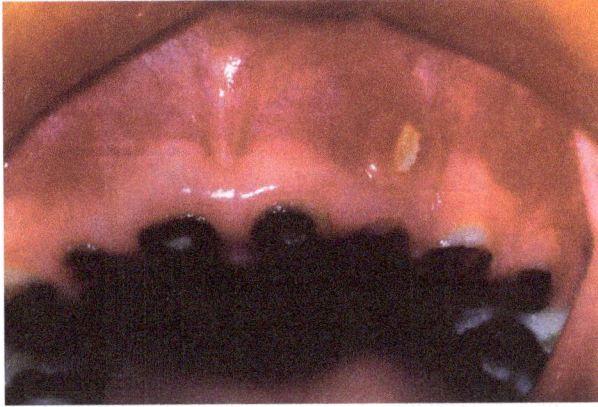

Figure 5. Radix relicta and bone penetration

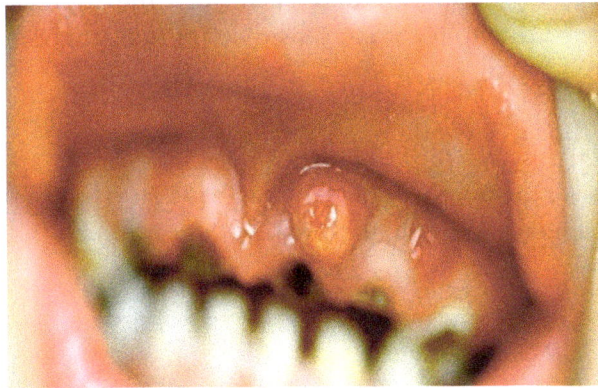

Figure 6. Abscess and fistula

Local situation – the gingiva is edematic, hyperemic and under pressure it is painful. Also while applying a slightly harder pressure from the gingival pocket purulent secret will come out. The tooth is extremely sensitive to palpation and percussion. (Fig.7)

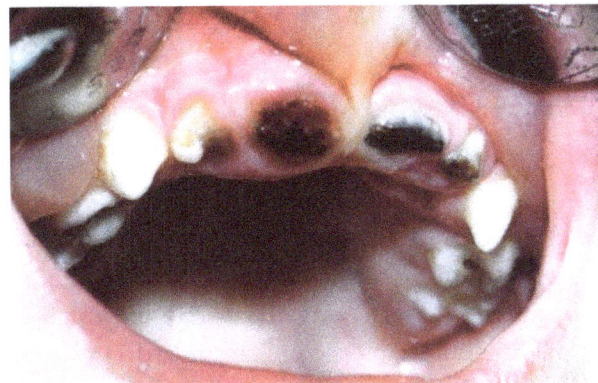

Figure 7. Edematic and hyperemic gingiva

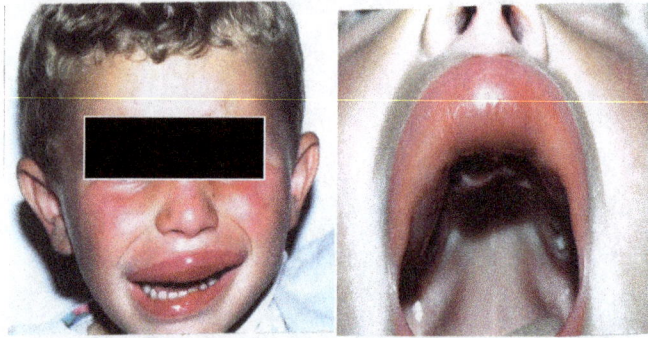

Figure 8. Spread of infection- result of ECC complications

General condition - pain, elevated temperature, fever, loss of appetite, the patient is pale and frightened. The patient cannot be fed as a result of edema of the lip and the gum inflammation. The food intake is affected due to the great sensitivity of the gangrenous roots in the upper front. (Fig.8)

Dental eruption disorders as a result of the remaining roots

As a result of root persistence, among others, it may have an effect in the eruption disorders of permanent teeth causing orthodontic abnormality (Fig. 9, 10.)

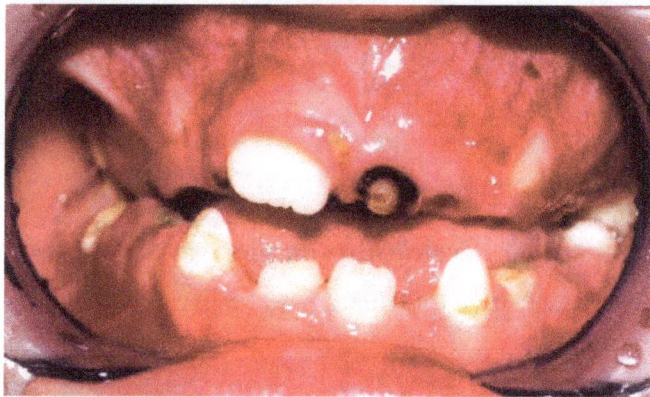

Figure 9. Persistence of radix relicta and disorders of permanent tooth eruption

Early Extraction

Consequence of an early childhood caries is the "loss" or extraction of teeth (Figure 11 & 12). Extraction of the teeth is approved when the clinical conditions become more serious, as a result of complications. But also: extraction may be due to unprofessional interference from the insisting parent, and the acceptance by the physician to do the extraction. The extraction, for example may be serial if it is decided by the therapist.

Consequences of Early extraction can be:

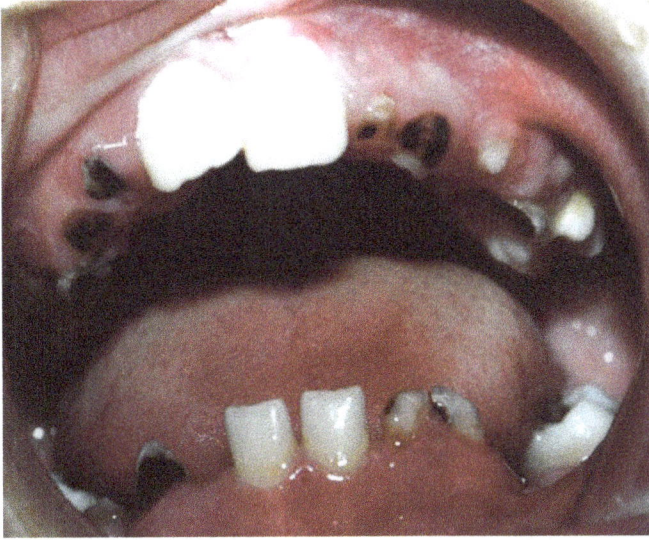

Figure 10. Orthodontic abnormality-result of radix relicta persistence

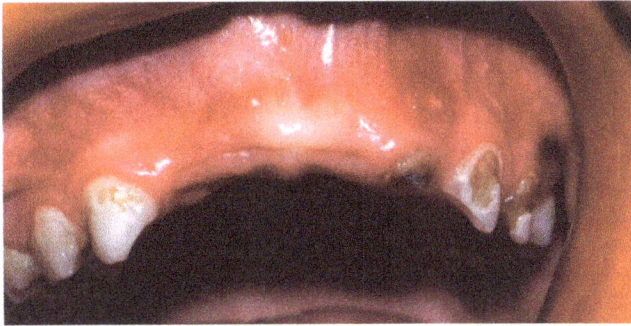

Figure 11. Early extraction of teeth

- abnormalities in the tooth eruption,

- speech impediment (incorrect pronunciation of letters),

- barriers in eating, poor aesthetics, etc.

Avoidance of these effects is done by prosthetic work, whose role would be: space mainte-nance, the normal pronunciation of letters, aesthetic improvement, etc.

5. Discussion

- *Risk factors of ECC*

Considering the data from the literature, the role of S mutans in the etiology of ECC, especially in the initial phase, is very crucial. These data also demonstrate the high prevalence of this

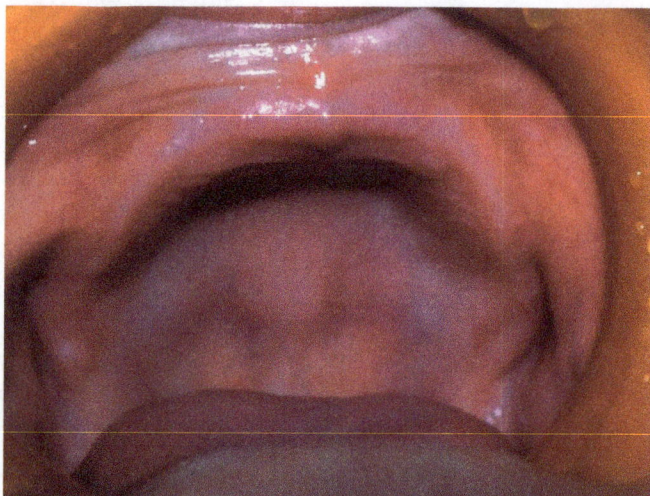

Figure 12. Total extraction of teeth-result of ECC complications

bacterium in preschool children. S mutans is found at the earliest ages, with the prevalence of 53% in 6- to 12-month-old children (Milgrom 2000), 60% in 15-month-olds (Karn 1998), 67% in 18-month-old Swedes (Hallonsten et al. 1995), and 94.7% in 3- to 4-year-old Chinese (Li et al. 1994). Almost all preschool urban Icelandic children were found to carry S mutans (Holbrook 1993). According to the studies of Ge and Caufield, all S-ECC children were S mutans–positive (Ge 2008). Borutta 2002, found that in 80% of children (3 years old) diagnosed with caries, the presence of S mutans was demonstrated, while higher counts of this bacterium were found in children with ECC.

The high prevalence of S mutans was also demonstrated in our study: 98% of preschool children. Expressed in colony-forming units (CFU/mL saliva), 93% of the ECC children in our study had a high S. mutans counts (CFU > 10^5). Higher salivary counts of *S. mutans* have been correlated with high dmft values (11.5) in our study. This significant correlation between high dmft or caries experience and high S mutans counts has been demonstrated in other studies (Köhler et al. 1995, Twetman & Frostner 1991, Maciel 2001).

In our study, the sweets consumption of children with ECC was very high. Almost 4/5 of ECC children have sweet snacks more than twice a day. It is of great concern that kindergartens as educational institutions do not have a more serious approach to a healthy diet and reduction of sugary food. On the contrary, at least once a day, sweet food (jam, chocolate, cream, biscuits, or cake) is served to children. Also, serving of this food is very common between meals. The literature also shows a high consumption of sweets between meals (Ölmez 2003) and high caries values in children who have frequent sweets (Holbrook 1989).

Another important factor in the etiology of ECC is bottle feeding, which is accompanied by high salivary counts of *S mutans*. The relationship between bottle usage and salivary counts of S mutans (Mohan 1998) has been reported. In the children that were in the study, the duration of bottle feeding with sweetened milk or juice was very long, wherein nearly 4/5 of children were bottle fed from 1 to 3 and more years.

Another harmful practice is putting children to sleep with a juice-filled bottle, which is practiced in 2/3 of children with ECC, although Johnsen has reported that 78% of parents of children with ECC had attempted to substitute water for a cariogenic liquid (e.g., apple juice, formula) in the bedtime nursing bottle [Johnsen]. A review of the literature from the etiological point of view of ECC shows that "the use of a bottle at night" is not the only cause of ECC (Plat 2000).

Oral hygiene habits established at the age of 1 can be maintained throughout early childhood (Wendt 1995). There is a high level of negligence in the oral hygiene of our children. More than half do not brush their teeth at all, exhibiting a very high oral hygiene index-OHI (1.52). The importance of the primary dentition of oral health promotion must be focused on the education of mothers to motivate their children for oral hygiene. Unfortunately, we found "bad conviction" of mothers regarding primary teeth that they will be replaced, thus neglecting the care for children's teeth. Data from the literature show that cooperation of mothers is very important in overcoming the belief that the deciduous dentition can be neglected (Rosamund 2003).

Mothers' knowledge and behaviours of oral hygiene are the key components for children's oral health care. The child imitates parental behaviours, including oral hygiene habits; thus, tooth brushing at an early age depends on maternal knowledge and behaviours. In our study, 38% of the mothers stated that their children did not brush their teeth at all. Only 11% of the interviewed mothers demonstrated proper techniques of tooth brushing. Unfortunately, a relatively low percentage of mothers (24%) stated that tooth brushing should last at least 2 to 3 minutes. The interviewed mothers rarely assisted their children during tooth brushing (5%).Even though fluoride and antimicrobial agents have a beneficial role in preventing caries, an insignificant number of interviewed mothers stated that they had knowledge regarding fluoride and they did not practice these preventive methods with their children (Begzati et al. 2014).

Besides fluoride treatments, an antimicrobial treatment option has become a serious consideration for many dental professionals. The data from the literature have confirmed the positive antibacterial role of chlorhexidine in the destruction of S. mutans colonies and inhibiting caries (Featherstone 2004, Zhang et al. 2006).

From the answers of mothers concerning fluoride use, we ascertained a marked lack of knowledge about the benefits of this agent in maintaining healthy tooth structure. This information gap can be inferred from their answers. When asked, "Do you give fluoride tablets to your child?" their answers were stated as if they have been asked about some medication: "I give those tablets to my child as needed." The absence of fluoride in Kosovo's municipal drinking water may highly influence caries prevalence rates in children.

Nutritional counseling, fluoride therapy, and oral hygiene may be required to prevent development of carious lesions in children. In the case of high-risk patients such as ECC children with a predominance of high salivary counts of S mutans, the use of either the antibacterial rinse chlorhexidine gluconate or the oral health care gel chlorhexidine has been suggested (Featherstone 2004).

The oral health promotion and preventive measures are also influenced by social and economic factors. Statistical data from Kosovo are as follows: large families (with average size of 6.5 members), high unemployment rate (in 2008 it marked 45.4%, for female 56.4%), high birth rate (16%) and the lowest economic growth in the region [56], represent some of the aggravating factors when dealing with the health issues of the population, including oral health issues (Ministry of Public Administration. Statistical Office of Kosovo 2010).

Given the complexity of factors associated with ECC, it is unfortunate that most of the interest has only been from dental organizations. The critical change needed to accomplish the necessary research related to prevention of ECC is to expand our network through inclusion other health professionals, community leaders, national organizations serving children, and political leaders (Ismaili 1998).

- *Consequences of ECC*

Scientific research suggests that the development of ECC occurs in 3 stages. The first stage is characterized by a primary infection of the oral cavity with ECC. The second stage is the proliferation of these organisms to pathogenic levels as a consequence of frequent and prolonged exposure to cariogenic substrates. Finally, a rapid demineralization and cavitation of the enamel occurs, resulting in rampant dental caries (Wyne 1998). A 1-year follow-up of ECC development from the initial stage, representing decay at the enamel level and its progression to more destructive stages, shows even development in all affected teeth. It is quite an acute development, because in 2/3 of the children, the ECC has progressed to more complicated stages (destructive and radix relicta stages). Within 1 year, the dmft values have increased to 3.7. Consecutively, these children commonly experience pain from pulpitis, gangrene, and apical periodontitis. Also, these conditions are often followed by abscesses and cellulitis, sometimes with phlegmona, seriously endangering the child's general health. De Grauwe, in describing the progression of ECC, has noticed that the development of caries from the enamel to the dentin level can occur within 6 months (De Grauwe et al. 2004). The rapid development of ECC and its clinical appearance, especially in primary incisors, identifies it in its initial stages as a risk factor for future caries in the primary and permanent dentitions (Al-Shalan et al. 1997).

Children with congenital heart anomalies are frequent patients in our departments, some of them exhibiting severe ECC. There is strong evidence that untreated dental disease is an important etiological factor in the pathogenesis of infective endocarditis, a condition that still carries a high risk of mortality (Child 1996).

Preventive measures for ECC (Begzati et al. 2012)

Early childhood caries (ECC) is a health problem with biological, social and behavioral determinants. Intervention treatment does not resolve this problem. It is difficult, sometimes impossible and expensive.

The only safest way is prevention of this complex pathology. European Academy of Pediatric Dentistry (2008) has recommended general strategies for ECC prevention:

- Oral health assessments with counseling at regularly scheduled visits during the first year of life are an important strategy to prevent ECC

- Children's teeth should be brushed daily with a smear of fluoride toothpaste as soon as they erupt

- Professional applications of fluoride varnish are recommended at least twice yearly in groups or individuals at risk.

- Parents of infants and toddlers should be encouraged to reduce behaviours that promote the early transmission of mutans streptococci.

Based on these recommendations, we will describe detailed preventive measures: primary prevention – prenatal and postnatal care; and secondary prevention – parents' and dental professionals' role.

- **Primary prevention**

It should begin during prenatal period and it consists of pregnant woman's needs' fulfillment with necessary and healthy products;

Proper quality of food for the newborn during the enamel maturation phase;

Fluoridation of newly-erupted teeth;

Antimicrobial therapy with chlorhexidine.

- **Secondary prevention**

Mothers' education on recognizing the first signs of ECC using "lift-the-lip" technique. The aim of this measure is early detection of the so-called "white spot".

Parents should be encouraged to avoid bad feeding habits of their children and give effort for proper feeding:

- breast-feeding of the baby;
- the use of cup instead of the bottle as early as possible;
- not sleeping with bottle in mouth;
- avoid the use of fabricated juices or soda;
- the use of natural, a little sweetened, juice or tea, or just water;
- avoid the discontinuation of bottle use by the method "bottle is gone";
- reduce the liquid in the bottle, gradually by night,
- reduce sweets as much as possible;
- no sweets between meals;
- daily tooth brushing, at least twice a day, obligatory before going to bed.

Necessary consultations with the dentist -

Professional education activity targeting primary care health providers (pediatricians, internists, family physicians, obstetricians, mid-level medical practitioners):

- early identification of disease,

- fluoride supplements as appropriate,

- healthful feeding practices,

- snacking behaviors that promote good oral health, and

- referral to the dentist by 12 months of age.

6. Conclusions

Oral health is integral to general health and should not be considered in isolation. Oral diseases have detrimental effects on an individual's physical and psychological well-being and reduce quality of life. The commonest disease is dental caries. Caries progression or reversal is determined by the balance between protective and pathological factors in the mouth. The most important component in the treatment of the caries disease is prevention. Understanding the balance between pathological factors and protective factors is the key to successful prevention of caries. Analyzing the etiology, prevalence, clinical specifics, consequences and complications, caries in general and ECC in particular are estimated as serious diseases, which represent not only health problem, but also a great serious social and economic problem.

Consequence of an early childhood caries, especially in underdeveloped countries, can be very severe, spanning from tooth loss to general health disorders. One of the complications of untreated ECC is the "loss" or extraction of teeth. Consequences of early extraction can be: abnormalities in the tooth eruption, speech impediment (incorrect pronunciation of letters), barriers in eating, poor aesthetics, etc.

The rapid development of ECC, especially in primary incisors, identifies it in its initial stages as a risk factor for future caries in the primary and permanent dentitions. There is strong evidence that untreated dental disease is an important etiological factor in the pathogenesis of infective endocarditis, a condition that still carries a high risk of mortality.

The risk factors for early childhood caries include a number of social and behavioural determinants.

Primary prevention must start in the prenatal stage to fulfill the needs of pregnancy. Parents should be encouraged to avoid bad feeding habits and to instruct and supervise their children in tooth brushing. Mothers should be instructed to use the lift-the-lip technique to spot the white-spot lesions as first signs of dental caries. Newly erupted teeth must be treated with fluoride agents, and, as needed, antimicrobial agents containing chlorhexidine and thymol. Further investigation is needed to assess the effectiveness of new intervention strategies beyond traditional measures that are not strictly dependent on access to dental professional providers.

Permanent and sustained oral health promotion organized with the participation of the entire civil society, with the mandatory presence of key stakeholders in the areas of education and healthcare, represent one of the highest priorities. The WHO strategies and objectives implementation regarding oral health promotion should be understood in the right manner and should be implemented continuously.

Author details

Agim Begzati[1*], Merita Berisha[3], Shefqet Mrasori[2], Blerta Xhemajli-Latifi[1], Rina Prokshi[1], Fehim Haliti[1], Valmira Maxhuni[1], Vala Hysenaj-Hoxha[1] and Vlera Halimi[1]

*Address all correspondence to: agimbegzati@yahoo.com

1 Department of Pedodontics and Preventive Dentistry, School of Dentistry, Medical Faculty, University of Prishtina, Prishtina, Republic of Kosovo

2 Department of Endodnintic, Medical Faculty, University of Prishtina, Prishtina, Republic of Kosovo

3 National Institute of Public Health of Kosovo, Department of Social Medicine, Medical Faculty, University of Prishtina, Prishtina, Republic of Kosovo

References

[1] Arkin, E.B. (1986). The Healthy Mothers, Healthy Babies Coalition: four years of progress. *Public Health Repository*, Vol. 101, pp. 147-156.

[2] Acs, G., Shulman, R., Wai, M. & Chussid' S. (1999). The effect of dental rehabilitation on the body weight of children with early childhood caries. *Pediatric Dentistry*, Vol. 21, pp.109-113.

[3] Acs, G., Lodolini, G., Kaminsky, S. & Cisneros, G.J.(1992). Effect of nursing caries on body weight in a pediatric population. *Pediatric Dentistry*, Vol. 14, pp:302-305.

[4] Al-Dashti, A.A., Williams, S.A. & Curzon, M.E.(1995). Breast feeding, bottle feeding and dental caries in Kuwait, a country with low-fluoride levels in the water supply. *Community Dental Health*. Vol.12, pp.42–47.

[5] Apostolova, D., Asprovsa, V. & Simovska N (2003). Circular caries-ECC-a problem at the earliest age. *8th Congress of the Balkan Stomatological Society*, (Abstract Book) Tirana, 2003.

[6] Al-Shalan, T.A., Erickson, P.R. & Hardie, N.A.(1997). Primary incisor decay before age 4 as a risk factor for future dental caries. *Paediatric Dentistry*,Vol.19, No.1, pp. 37-41.

[7] Begzati, A., Meqa, K., Siegenthaler, D., Berisha, M. & Mautsch, W. (2011). Dental health evaluation of children in Kosovo. *European Journal of Dentistry*, Vol. 5, pp. 32-39

[8] Begzati, A., Bytyci, A., Meqa, K., Latifi-Xhemajli, B. & Berisha, M. (2014). Mothers' Behaviours and Knowledge Related to Caries Experience of Their Children, *Oral Health & Preventive Dentistry*, Vol.2, pp.133-140

[9] Begzati, A., Meqa, K. & Berisha, M. Early childhood caries in preschool children of Kosovo - a serious public health problem . *BMC Public Health* 2010, 10:788

[10] Begzati, A., K. Meqa, K., Azemi, M., Begzati, Aj., Kutllovci, T., Xhemajli, B. & Berisha, M.(2012) Oral health care in children - a preventive perspective, In: *Oral health Care-Pediatric, Research, Epidemiology and Clinical Practices*, Published by InTech, 2012; 19-59.

[11] Bruered, B., Kinney, M.B. & Bothwell, E. (1989). Preventing baby bottle tooth decay in American Indian and Alaska native communities: a model for planning. *Public Health Repository*, Vol. 104, No. 6, pp. 631-640.

[12] Beltrami, G.(1952) .Black teeth in toddlers. Siècle Medical 1932 Apr 4. Cited in Beltrami, G. *La mélanodontie infantile* . Marseilles, By Leconte Editeur.

[13] Berkowitz. R.J., Turner, J. & Green, P. (1980). Primary oral infection of infants with Streptococcus mutans. *Archives of Oral Biology*, Vol. 25, pp. 221-224.

[14] Barbakov. F., Scheil. W. & Imfel, T.(1985). Observations of SnF2-treated Human Enamel Using the Scanning Electron microscope, *Journal of Dentistry for Children*, Vol.52, pp.279-287.

[15] Berkowitz, R.J. (1996). Etiology of nursing caries; a microbiologic perspective. *Journal of Public Health Dentistry*, Vol. 56, No. 1, pp. 51-54.

[16] Berkowitz, R.J., Jordan, H.V. & White, G. (1975). The early establishment of Streptococcus mutans in the mouths of infants. *Archives of Oral Biology*, Vol.20, pp.171-174.

[17] Burne, R.A.(1998). Oral streptococci products of their environment, *Journal of Dental Research*, Vol.77, pp.445-452.

[18] Borutta, A., Kneist, S. & Eherler, D.P. (2002). Oral health and Occurrence of Salivary S. mutans in Small Children, *Journal of Dental and Oral Medicine*, Vol. 4, No. 3, Poster 128.

[19] Berkowitz, R.J., Turner, J. & Green P.(1981). Maternal salivary levels of Streptococcus mutans: The primary oral infection in infants. *Archives of Oral Biology*, Vol.26, pp. 147-149.

[20] Carlsson, P.(1989). Distribution of mutans streptococci in populations with different levels of sugar consumption. *Scandinavian journal of dental research*, Vol.97 No.2, pp. 120-125.

[21] Centers for Disease Control and Prevention (CDCP), conference. Atlanta, GA, September 1994.

[22] Caufield, P.W., Cutter, G.R. & Dasanayake A.P.(1993). Initial acquisition of mutans streptococci by infants: evidence for a discrete window of infectivity. *Journal of Dental Research*, Vol.72, pp. 37-45.

[23] Catalanotto, F.A., Shklair, I.I. & Keene, H.J.(1975). Prevalence and localization of Streptococcus mutans in infants and children. *Journal of the American Dental Association*, Vol.91, pp:606-609.

[24] Child, J.S. (1996). Risks for and prevention of infective endocarditis. In: Child JS, ed. *Cardiology Clinics—Diagnosis and Management of Infective Endocarditis.* Philadelphia, Pa: WB Saunders Co, Vol. 14, pp. 327-343.

[25] Drury, Th.F., Horowitz, A.M., Ismail, A.I., Maertens, M.P., Rozier, R.G. & Selwitz, R.H. (1999). Diagnosing and reporting Early Childhood Caries for Research Purposes. *Journal of Public Health Dentistry*, Vol. 59, pp. 192-197.

[26] Davis, G.N. (1998). Early childhood caries-a synopsis. *Community Dentistry and Oral Epidemiology*,Munksgaard , Vol. 26, pp.106-116.

[27] Derkson, G.D. & Ponti, P. (1982). Nursing bottle syndrome: prevalence end etiology in a non fluoridated city. *Journal of the Canadian Dental Association*, Vol. 6, pp. 389-393.

[28] Douglass, J.M., Douglass, A.B. & Silk HJ.(2004). A practical guide to infant oral health. *Am Fam Physician*. Vol.70, pp.2113–2120.

[29] Elice, C.E. & Fields, C.W.(1990). Failure to thrive: Rewire of literature, case reports and implications for dental treatment. *Pediatric Dentistry*, Vol.12, pp.185-189.

[30] European Academy of Paediatric Dentistry (EAPD 2008). *Guidelines on Prevention of Early Childhood Caries: An EAPD Policy Document.* Dublin, Ireland.

[31] Featherstone, J.D.B. (2004). The Caries Balance: The Basis for Caries Management by Risk Assessment. *Oral Health and Preventive Dentistry*, Vol. 2, No 1, pp. 259-264

[32] Fass, E.(1962). Is bottle feeding of milk a factor in dental caries? *Journal of Dentistry for Children* Vol.29, pp. 245-251.

[33] Fédération Dentaire Internationale –FDI(1988). Technical report No. 31. Review of methods of identification of high caries groups and individuals. *International Dental Journal, Vol.*38, pp. 177-189.

[34] Ge. Y., Caufield, P.W., Fisch, G.S. & Li. Y.(2008). Streptococcus mutans and Strepto-coccus sanguinis Colonization Correlated with Caries Experience in Children. *Caries Res,* Vol.42, pp.444-448.

[35] De Grauwe, A., Aps, J.K. & Martens, L.C. (2004). Early Childhood Caries (ECC): What's in a name? *European Journal of Pediatric Dentistry,* Vol. 5, No. 2, pp. 62-70.

[36] Goose, D.H.(1967). Infant Feeding and Caries of the Incisors: an epidemiological Ap-proach. *Caries Research,* Vol.1 , pp.167-173.

[37] Galdvin, M. & Trattler, B.(2004) Clinical Microbiology, MedMaster, Inc., Miami, Flor-ida-USA.

[38] Horowitz, H.S.(1998). Research issues in early childhood caries. *Community Dentistry and Oral Epidemiology, Vol.*17, pp. 292-295.

[39] Hamada, S. & Slade, H.D.(1980). Biology, immunology and Cariogencity of Strepto-coccus mutans; *Microbiology Reviews,* Vol.44, pp. 331-384.

[40] Harris, O.N. & Garsia, F. (1999). Primary Preventive Dentistry, by Applenton & Lange, Stamford.

[41] Holt, R.D., Winter, G.B., Downer, M.C. & Bellis, W.J. (1996). Caries in pre-school chil-dren in Camden 1993/94. *British Dental Journal,* Vol. 181, pp. 405-410.

[42] Hunt, R.J. (1986). Percent agreement, Pearson's correlation, and kappa as measures of inter-examiner reliability. *Journal of Dental Research,* Vol. 65, pp.128-130

[43] Hallonsten, A.L., Wendt, L.K., Mejar, I., Birkhed, D., Hakansson, C., Lindwall, A.M., Edwardsson, S., Koch, G. (1995). Dental Caries and prolonged breast-feeding in 18-month- old. Swedish children. *International Journal of Paediatric Dentistry,* Vol.5, No.3, pp.149-155.

[44] Holbrook, W.P.(1993). Dental caries and cariogenic factors in pre-school urban Ice-landic children. *Caries Res,*Vol. 27, No.5, pp.431-437.

[45] Holbrook, W.P., Kristinsson, M.J., Gunnarsdóttir, S. & Briem, B. (1989). Caries preva-lence, Streptococcus mutans and sugar intake among 4-year-old urban children in Iceland. *Community Dentistry and Oral Epidemiology,* Vol. 17, No. 6, pp. 292-295.

[46] Harper, D.S. & Loesche, W.J.(1984). Growth and acid tolerance of human dental pla-que bacteria. *Archives of Oral Biology,* Vol. 29, pp.843-848.

[47] Huseinbegović, A. (2001). Social and medical aspects of primary dentition caries in urban conditions. Master degree- Sarajevo.

[48] Horowitz, H.S. (1998). Research issues in early childhood caries. *Community Dentistry and Oral Epidemiology,* Vol. 26, No. 1, pp. 67-81.

[49] Ismail, A.I. & Sohn, W. (1999). A Systematic Review of Clinical Diagnostic Criteria of Early Childhood Caries. *Journal of Public Health Dentistry,* Vol. 59, No. 3, pp. 171-191.

[50] Ismail, A.I. (1998). Prevention of early childhood caries. *Community Dentistry and Oral Epidemiology*, Vol. 26, No.1, pp. 49-61.

[51] Johnsen, D.C. (1982). Characteristics and backgrounds of children with "nursing caries." *Pediatric Dentistry*, Vol. 4, No. 3, pp. 218–224.

[52] Jacobi, A. (1862). Dentition. *Its Derangements. A Course of Lectures Delivered in the New York Medical College.* New York: Ballière Brothers

[53] James, P.M.C., Parfitt, G.J. & Falkner, F. (1957). A study of the aetiology of labial caries of the deciduous incisor teeth in small children. *British Dental Journal*, Vol. 103, No. 2, pp.37–40.

[54] Kobaslia, S., Maglaic, N. & Begovic, A. (2000). Caries prevalence of Sarajevo children. *Acta Stomatologica Croatica*, Vol. 34, pp. 83-85

[55] Konig, K.G. & Navia, E.M. (1995). Nutritional role of sugars in oral health. *American Journal of Clinical Nutrition*, Vol. 62, Suppl. pp. 275S-83S.

[56] Keyes, P.H.(1962). Recent advances in dental caries research. *International Dental Journal, Vol.* 12, pp. 443-464.

[57] Kaste, L.M. & Gift, H.C. (1995). Inappropriate infant bottle feeding: Status of the Healthy People 2000 Objective. *Archives of Pediatrics & Adolescent Medicine.* Vol. 149, pp.786-791.

[58] Kaste, L.M., Selwitz, R.H., Oldakowski, R.J., Brunelle, J.A., Win, D.M. & Brown, L.J. (1996). Coronal Caries in the Primary and Permanent Dentition of Children and Adolescents 1-17 Years of Age: United States, 1988-1991, *Journal of Dental Research,*Vol. 75, pp. 631-641.

[59] Karn, T.A., O'Sullivan, D.M. & Tinannoff N. (1988). Colonization of mutans streptococci in 8- to 15- month-old children. *Journal of Public Health Dentistry,,* Vol. 58, No.3. pp. 248-249.

[60] Köhler, B., Andreen, I. & Jonsson, B. (1988). The earlier the colonization by mutans streptococci, the higher the caries prevalence at 4 years of age. *Oral Microbiology and Immunology*, Vol. 3, pp. 14-17.

[61] Köhler, B., Bjarnason, S., Care, R., Mackevica, I. & Rence, I. (1995). Mutans streptococci and dental caries prevalence in a group of Latvian preschool children. *European Journal of Oral Sciences*, Vol. 103, No. 4, pp. 264-266.

[62] Koga, T., Asakawa, H., Okahashi, N. & Hamada, S.(1986). Sucrose –dependent cell adherence and cariogenicity of serotype-c streptococcus mutans *Journal of general microbiology,* . Vol.132, pp.2873-2883.

[63] Lopez, L., Berkowitz, R.J., Moss, M.E. & Weinstein, P. (2000). Mutans streptotocci prevalence in Puerto Rican babies with cariogenic feeding behaviors. *Pediatric Dentistry*, Vol. 22, No. 4, pp. 299–301.

[64] Li, Y., Navia, J.M. & Caufield, P.W.(1994). Colonization by mutans streptococci in mouths of 3- and 4- year -old Chinese children with or without enamel hypoplasia. *Archives of Oral Biology,* , Vol.39, N.12, pp.1057-1062.

[65] Loesche, W.J.(1986). Role of Streptococcus mutans in human dental decay; *Microbiological reviews,* Vol.50, pp. 353-380.

[66] Maciel, S.M., Marcenes, W. & Sheiham, A. (2001). The relationship between sweetness preference, levels of salivary mutans streptococci and caries experience in Brazilian pre-school children. *International Journal of Paediatric Dentistry,* Vol. 11, pp. 123-130.

[67] Mohan, A.M., O'Sallivan, D.M. & Tinanoff, N. (1998). The relationship between bottle usage/content, age and number of teeth with mutans streptococci colonization in 6-24 – month-old children. *Community Dentistry and Oral Epidemiology* Vol. 26, Suppl. 1, pp. 12-20.

[68] Ministry of Public Administration. Statistical Office of Kosovo. (http://esk.rks-ov.net/eng/index.php? option=com_docman&task=doc_download&gid=870&Item-id=8). Accessed on October 20th, 2010.

[69] Marthaler, M., O'Mullane, M. & Vrbic, V. (1996). The prevalence of dental caries in Europe 1990-1995. *Caries Research,* Vol. 30, pp. 237-255

[70] Marković, M.(1976). Etiologija malokluzija-book. Beograd, pp. 141-171

[71] Milgrom, P., Riedy, C.A., Weinstein, P., Tanner, A.C., Manibusan, L.& Bruss J(2000). Dental caries and its relationship to bacterial infection, hypoplasia, diet, and oral hygiene in 6- to 36-month-old children. *Community Dent Oral Epidemiol,* Vol. 28, pp: 295-306.

[72] Mcdonald, R. & Avery, D.A.(2000). Dentistry for the Child and Adolescent, Mosby.

[73] Norman, O.H. & Franklin, G. (1999). *Primary Preventive Dentistry.* Appleton & Lange, Stamford, Connecticut.

[74] O'Sullivan, D.M. & Tinanoff, N. (1993). Social and biological factors contributing to caries of the maxillary anterior teeth. *Pediatric Dentistry,* Vol. 15, pp. 41-44.

[75] Ölmez, S., Uzamis, M. & Erdem, G. (2003). Association between early childhood caries and clinical, microbiological, oral hygiene and dietary variables in rural Turkish children. *The Turkish Journal of Pediatrics,* Vol. 45, pp. 231-236.

[76] Plat, L. & Cebazas, M.C. (2000). Early childhood dental caries. Building community system for young children. Los Angeles, CA: University of California-Los Angeles Center for Healthier Children, Families and Communities, Vol. 32, exec. summ. (4 pp.).

[77] Petti, S., Iannazzo, S., Gemelli, G., Rocchi, R., Novello, M.R., Ortensi, V., Nicolussi, A., Simonetti D'Arca, A. & Tarsitani, G. (2001). Incidence of caries in a sample of 3-7-

year old children in Rome who were not included in population prevention programs. Ann Ig. Vol.13, No.4, pp.329-38.

[78] Quartey, J.B. & Williamson, D.D.(1998). Prevalence of early childhood caries at Harris County clinics. *Journal of Dentistry for Children. Vol.* 7, pp.127-131.

[79] Raiç, Z.(1985). Deçija i preventivna stomatologija-book, Zagreb.

[80] Reisine, S., Douglass, J.M. (1998). Psychosocial and behavioral issues in early childhood caries. *Community Dentistry and Oral Epidemiology*; Vol. 26, No.1, pp. 32-44.

[81] Rosamund, L.H. & Tracy, W. (2003). An oral health promotion program for an urban minority population of preschool children. *Community Dentistry and Oral Epidemiolology*, Vol. 31, No. 5, pp. 392-399.

[82] Russell, R.(2003). Microbiological aspects of caries prevention, Prevention of oral disease, Oxford.

[83] Ripa, L.W. (1988). Nursing caries: a comprehensive review. *Pediatric Dentistry*, Vol. 10, pp. 268-282.

[84] Soames, J.V. & Southam, J.C. (1999). Oral Pathology-book, by Oxford University press.

[85] Stile, H.M., Loesche, W.J. & O'Brien T.C. (1976). Microbial Aspects of Dental Caries. London, England: Information Retrieval; Vol. 1. pp:187-199.

[86] Schroth, R.J., Brothwell, D.J. & Moffatt, M.E.K.(2007). Caregiver knowledge and attitudes of preschool oral health and early childhood caries (ECC). *International Journal of Circumpolar Health* Vol. 66, pp. 153-167.

[87] Stosiç, P.(1991). Deçja i preventivna stomatologija-book. Beograd.

[88] Soames, J.V. & Southam, J.C. (1999). Oral Pathology. 3rd ed. Oxford

[89] Seow, W.K.(1998). Biological mechanisms of early childhood caries. *Community Dentistry and Oral Epidemiology, Vol.* 26, pp. 8-27.

[90] Tinanoff, N., Kaste, L.M. & Corbin, S.B. (1998). Early childhood caries: a positive beginning. *Community Dentistry and Oral Epidemiolology*, Vol. 26, No. 1, pp. 117-119.

[91] Twetman, S. & Frostner, N. (1991). Salivary mutans streptococci and caries prevalence in 8-year-old Swedish schoolchildren. *Swedish Dental Journal*, Vol. 15, No. 3, pp. 145-151.

[92] Tanner, ACR.(2002). The microbiota of young children from tooth and tongue samples. *Journal of Dental Research,* Vol.81, pp:53-57.

[93] Thomas, F.D., Alice, M.H., Amidi, I.I., Marco, P.M., Rozier, G.R. & Robert, H.(1999). Diagnosing and Reporting Early Childhood Caries for Research Purposes, *Journal of Public Health Dentistry*, Vol.59, pp.192-197.

[94] Thomas, A.K., David, M.O. & Norman, T.(1998). Colonization of Mutans Streptococci in 8 to 15 month-old Children. *Journal of Public Health Dentistry,* Vol.58, pp:248-249.

[95] Tsai, I.A., Johnsen, C.D., Lin, Y. & Kuang-Hung, H.(2001). A study of risk factors associated with nursing caries in Taiwanes children aged 24-48 months. *International Journal of Pediatric Dentistry,* Vol.11, pp.147-149.

[96] US Department of Health and Human Services. (2000). *Oral Health in America*: A Report of the Surgeon General. Rockville, MD: US Department of Health and Human Services, National Institute of Dental and Craniofacial Research, National Institutes of Health.

[97] Wan, A.K.L.(2001). Oral colonization of *Streptococcus mutans* in six-month-old predentate Infants. *Journal of Dental Research,* Vol.12, pp.2060-2065.

[98] Wyne, A.H. (1999). Early chlidhood caries: nomenclatur and case definition. *Community Dentistry and Oral Epidemiology,* Vol. 7, pp. 313-315.

[99] Wendt, L.K. & Birkhed, D.(1995). Dietary habits related to caries development and immigrant status in infants and toddlers living in Sweden. *Acta Odontologica Scandinavica, Vol.*53, pp. 339-344.

[100] Wendt, L.K. (1995). On oral health in infants and toddlers. *Swedish Dental Journal,* Vol. 19, Suppl., pp. 106:1-62.

[101] Winter, G.B., Hamilton, M.C. & James, P.M.C. (1966). Role of comforter as en etiological factor in rampant caries of deciduous dentition. *Archives of Diseases in Children,* Vol. 417, pp. 207-212.

[102] Whiley, R.A., & Beighton, D.(2013) "Streptococci and Oral Streptococci." Bite-Sized Tutorials. N.p. Web. 2013 *https://microbewiki.kenyon.edu/index.php/Streptococcus_mutans-_Tooth_Decay_References*

[103] Wierzbicka, M., Carlsson, P., Struzycka, I., Iwanicka-Frankowska, E. & Bratthall, D. (1987). Oral health and factors related to oral health in Polish schoolchildren. *Community Dentistry and Oral Epidemiology,* Vol. 15, No. 4, pp.177-239.

[104] Wan, A.K.L., Seow, K.(2001). Association of Streptococcus mutans infection and oral developmental nodules in predentate infants. *Journal of Dental Research,* Vol.80, pp. 1945-1948.

Permissions

The contributors of this book come from diverse backgrounds, making this book a truly international effort. This book will bring forth new frontiers with its revolutionizing research information and detailed analysis of the nascent developments around the world.

We would like to thank all the contributing authors for lending their expertise to make the book truly unique. They have played a crucial role in the development of this book. Without their invaluable contributions this book wouldn't have been possible. They have made vital efforts to compile up to date information on the varied aspects of this subject to make this book a valuable addition to the collection of many professionals and students.

This book was conceptualized with the vision of imparting up-to-date information and advanced data in this field. To ensure the same, a matchless editorial board was set up. Every individual on the board went through rigorous rounds of assessment to prove their worth. After which they invested a large part of their time researching and compiling the most relevant data for our readers.

The editorial board has been involved in producing this book since its inception. They have spent rigorous hours researching and exploring the diverse topics which have resulted in the successful publishing of this book. They have passed on their knowledge of decades through this book. To expedite this challenging task, the publisher supported the team at every step. A small team of assistant editors was also appointed to further simplify the editing procedure and attain best results for the readers.

Apart from the editorial board, the designing team has also invested a significant amount of their time in understanding the subject and creating the most relevant covers. They scrutinized every image to scout for the most suitable representation of the subject and create an appropriate cover for the book.

The publishing team has been an ardent support to the editorial, designing and production team. Their endless efforts to recruit the best for this project, has resulted in the accomplishment of this book. They are a veteran in the field of academics and their pool of knowledge is as vast as their experience in printing. Their expertise and guidance has proved useful at every step. Their uncompromising quality standards have made this book an exceptional effort. Their encouragement from time to time has been an inspiration for everyone.

The publisher and the editorial board hope that this book will prove to be a valuable piece of knowledge for researchers, students, practitioners and scholars across the globe.

List of Contributors

Sanaa Alami, Hakima Aghoutan, Farid El Quars and Farid Bourzgui
Department of Dento-facial Orthopedic, Faculty of Dental Medicine, Hassan II University of Casablanca, Morocco

Samir Diouny
Chouaib Doukkali University, Faculty of Letters & Human Sciences, El Jadida, Morocco

Maen H. Zreaqat
Al-Ogaly Medical Group, Saudi Arabia

Javier de la Fuente Hernández, Fátima del Carmen Aguilar Díaz and María del Carmen Villanueva Vilchis
Escuela Nacional de Estudios Superiores, Unidad León. Universidad Nacional Autónomade México, México

Sergio Sánchez García
Unidad de Investigación en Epidemiología y Servicios de Salud. Área Envejecimiento. Centro Médico Nacional Siglo XXI. Instituto Mexicano del Seguro Social, México
Departamento de Salud Pública y Epidemiología Bucal. Facultad de Odontología. Universidad Nacional Autónoma de México, México

Erika Heredia Ponce
Departamento de Salud Pública y Epidemiología Bucal. Facultad de Odontología. Universidad Nacional Autónoma de México, México

Hisashi Fujita
Department of Bioanthropology, Niigata College of Nursing, Japan

Derek S J D'Souza
Pune, India

Preetika Chandna and Vivek K. Adlakha
Department of Paedodontics and Preventive Dentistry, Subharti Dental College, Meerut, Uttar Pradesh, India

Kristina Goršeta
Department of Pediatric and Preventive Dentistry, School of Dental Medicine, University of Zagreb, Croatia

Sukumaran Anil, Raed M. Alrowis and Hani S. AlMoharib
Department of Periodontics and Community Dentistry, College of Dentistry, King Saud University, Riyadh, Saudi Arabia

Elna P. Chalisserry
College of Dentistry, King Saud University, Riyadh, Saudi Arabia

Vemina P. Chalissery
Mahatma Gandhi Dental College and Hospital, Jaipur, Rajasthan, India

Asala F. Al-Sulaimani
King Saud University, Riyadh, Saudi Arabia

Agim Begzati, Blerta Xhemajli-Lati i, Rina Prokshi, Fehim Haliti, Valmira Maxhuni, Vala Hysenaj-Hoxha and Vlera Halimi
Department of Pedodontics and Preventive Dentistry, School of Dentistry, Medical Faculty, University of Prishtina, Prishtina, Republic of Kosovo

Shefqet Mrasori
Department of Endodnintic, Medical Faculty, University of Prishtina, Prishtina, Republic of Kosovo

Merita Berisha
National Institute of Public Health of Kosovo, Department of Social Medicine, Medical Faculty, University of Prishtina, Prishtina, Republic of Kosovo

Index